Sexual Health & STIs

Editor: Danielle Lobban

Volume 449

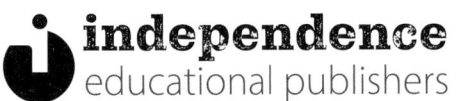

First published by Independence Educational Publishers

The Studio, High Green

Great Shelford

Cambridge CB22 5EG

England

© Independence 2024

Copyright

This book is sold subject to the condition that it shall not, by way of trade or otherwise, be lent, resold, hired out or otherwise circulated in any form of binding or cover other than that in which it is published without the publisher's prior consent.

Photocopy licence

The material in this book is protected by copyright. However, the purchaser is free to make multiple copies of particular articles for instructional purposes for immediate use within the purchasing institution. Making copies of the entire book is not permitted.

ISBN-13: 978 1 86168 909 2

Printed in Great Britain

Pureprint Group

Acknowledgements

The publisher is grateful for permission to reproduce the material in this book. While every care has been taken to trace and acknowledge copyright, the publisher tenders its apology for any accidental infringement or where copyright has proved untraceable. The publisher would be pleased to come to a suitable arrangement in any such case with the rightful owner.

The material reproduced in **issues** books is provided as an educational resource only. The views, opinions and information contained within reprinted material in **issues** books do not necessarily represent those of Independence Educational Publishers and its employees.

Although every effort has been made to ensure that website addresses are correct at time of going to press, Independence Educational Publishers cannot be held responsible for the content of any website mentioned in this book.

Images

Cover image courtesy of iStock. All other images courtesy of Freepik, Pixabay, Pexels, and Unsplash.

Additional acknowledgements

With thanks to the Independence team: Janey Hills, Klaudia Sommer and Jackie Staines.

Danielle Lobban

Cambridge, October 2024

Contents

Chapter 1: Sexual Health

What is sexual health?	1
The history of sexual health	2
Where can I get sexual health advice, now?	4
If I use a sexual health service will they tell my parents?	5
What happens at a sexual health check-up?	6
A comprehensive guide to smear tests	7
Genital hygiene	8
Consent	10
When is someone mentally ready to have sex?	12
How do I know if I am ready to have sex?	13
10 mega myths about sex	14

Chapter 2: Contraception

Why is contraception important?	15
Contraception and you	16
Where to get contraception	19
What should I do if a condom breaks or comes off?	20
Making informed decisions about taking the morning-after pill	21
Women in England to receive contraceptive pills at pharmacies	22

Chapter 3: STIs

What is an STI?	23
10 signs you may have a sexually transmitted infection (STI)	24
STIs: Get tested, get treated	25
Sexually transmitted infections found in 13-year-olds as cases hit record high	26
Guide to Sexually Transmitted Infections (STIs)	28
STI myths	30
HIV and AIDS: just the facts	31
What is HIV?	32
Myths about HIV	34
An HPV factsheet – everything you need to know	36
STIs through the centuries	39

Further Reading/Useful Websites	42
Glossary	43
Index	44

Introduction

Sexual Health & STIs is volume 449 in the **issues** series. The aim of the series is to offer current, diverse information about important issues in our world, from a UK perspective.

About *Sexual Health & STIs*

Sexual health is an issue that will always need open and honest discussion. This book explores contraception and STI prevention. It also looks at the importance of healthy, respectful relationships, the importance of more topical issues such as consent, sexting and safe online dating.

Our sources

Titles in the **issues** series are designed to function as educational resource books, providing a balanced overview of a specific subject.

The information in our books is comprised of facts, articles and opinions from many different sources, including:

- Newspaper reports and opinion pieces
- Website factsheets
- Magazine and journal articles
- Statistics and surveys
- Government reports
- Literature from special interest groups.

A note on critical evaluation

Because the information reprinted here is from a number of different sources, readers should bear in mind the origin of the text and whether the source is likely to have a particular bias when presenting information (or when conducting their research). It is hoped that, as you read about the many aspects of the issues explored in this book, you will critically evaluate the information presented.

It is important that you decide whether you are being presented with facts or opinions. Does the writer give a biased or unbiased report? If an opinion is being expressed, do you agree with the writer? Is there potential bias to the 'facts' or statistics behind an article?

Activities

Throughout this book, you will find a selection of assignments and activities designed to help you engage with the articles you have been reading and to explore your own opinions. Some tasks will take longer than others and there is a mixture of design, writing and research-based activities that you can complete alone or in a group.

Further research

At the end of each article we have listed its source and a website that you can visit if you would like to conduct your own research. Please remember to critically evaluate any sources that you consult and consider whether the information you are viewing is accurate and unbiased.

Issues Online

The **issues** series of books is complemented by our online resource, issuesonline.co.uk

On the Issues Online website you will find a wealth of information, covering over 75 topics, to support the PSHE and RSE curriculum.

Why Issues Online?

Researching a topic? Issues Online is the best place to start for...

Librarians

Issues Online is an essential tool for librarians: feel confident you are signposting safe, reliable, user-friendly online resources to students and teaching staff alike. We provide multi-user concurrent access, so no waiting around for another student to finish with a resource. Issues Online also provides FREE downloadable posters for your shelf/wall/table displays.

Teachers

Issues Online is an ideal resource for lesson planning, inspiring lively debate in class, and setting lessons and homework tasks.

Our accessible, engaging content helps deepen students' knowledge, promotes critical thinking, and develops independent learning skills.

Issues Online saves precious preparation time. We wade through the wealth of material on the internet to filter the best quality, most relevant and up-to-date information you need to start exploring a topic.

Our carefully selected, balanced content presents an overview and insight into each topic from a variety of sources and viewpoints.

Students

Issues Online is designed to support your studies in a broad range of topics, particularly social issues relevant to young people today.

There are thousands of articles, statistics and infographs instantly available to help you with homework, research, and assignments.

With 24/7 access using the powerful Algolia search system, you can find relevant information quickly, easily and safely anytime from your laptop, tablet or smartphone, in class or at home.

Visit issuesonline.co.uk to find out more!

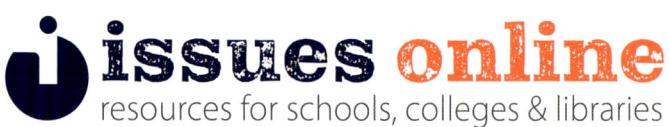

Chapter 1: Sexual Health

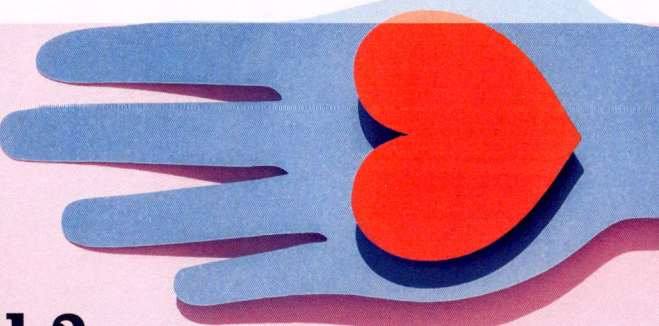

What is sexual health?

Sexual health is a broad term that encompasses various dimensions of our health and wellbeing related to sexuality. It involves more than just avoiding diseases or unplanned pregnancies; it's also about understanding and respecting your body, having safe and pleasurable sexual experiences, and navigating relationships in a healthy, respectful manner.

Understanding your body

At its core, sexual health starts with understanding and respecting your own body and desires. During the teenage years, many changes occur, both physically and emotionally. These changes are a normal part of growing up. It's important to learn about these changes, so you can understand what is happening to your body and feel comfortable with yourself.

Learning about your body isn't just about understanding how it works in a biological sense; it's also about recognising what feels good and what doesn't, knowing your limits, and being able to communicate those to others when the time is right. Remember, every person is unique, and there is a wide range of normal when it comes to physical development and desires.

Consent and communication

A crucial part of sexual health is understanding and practicing consent. Consent means agreeing to something, in this case, any form of sexual activity, freely and without pressure or being under the influence of substances. It's important that consent is enthusiastic, meaning everyone involved really wants to participate. Consent can also be withdrawn at any time, and if it is, all activities should stop immediately.

Good communication is essential for ensuring consent. It involves being able to express your own desires and limits clearly, and also listening to and respecting others' boundaries and feelings. Effective communication can help prevent misunderstandings and ensure that any sexual experience is positive for everyone involved.

Safe sex and avoiding sexually transmitted infections (STIs)

Another important aspect of sexual health is practicing safe sex to reduce the risk of sexually transmitted infections (STIs) and unwanted pregnancies. Safe sex practices include using condoms correctly every time you have sex, getting vaccinated against HPV, and undergoing regular sexual health check-ups. It's also about being informed and making responsible choices about your sexual health.

If you're sexually active or planning to be, it's important to educate yourself about STIs; how they're transmitted, how they can affect your health, and how to prevent them. Many STIs are asymptomatic, meaning they don't show any symptoms, so regular testing is crucial even if you feel fine.

Emotional aspects of sexual health

Sexual health is not just about physical health; it's also deeply connected to our emotional wellbeing. Healthy relationships, whether they're romantic, sexual, or platonic, are based on mutual respect, honesty, and care. Understanding and managing your emotions, as well as communicating effectively with partners about feelings and boundaries, are key skills for maintaining both your emotional wellbeing and sexual health.

Pressure from peers, partners, or society can make navigating sexual health challenging. Remember, it's okay to say no to anything you're not comfortable with, and it's okay to take your time to discover what you're comfortable with. Respecting your feelings and boundaries, and those of others, is a sign of strength and self-respect.

Conclusion

Sexual health is a vital part of overall health and wellbeing, especially during the teenage years when many people begin to explore their sexuality. It encompasses understanding your body and desires, practicing consent and communication, protecting yourself against STIs and unwanted pregnancies, and managing emotions in relationships. By being informed, respecting yourself and others, and practicing safe habits, you can navigate your sexual health with confidence and care.

Remember, being curious about your sexual health and seeking information is a sign of maturity. It shows that you're taking responsibility for your own wellbeing, which is a critical step towards adulthood.

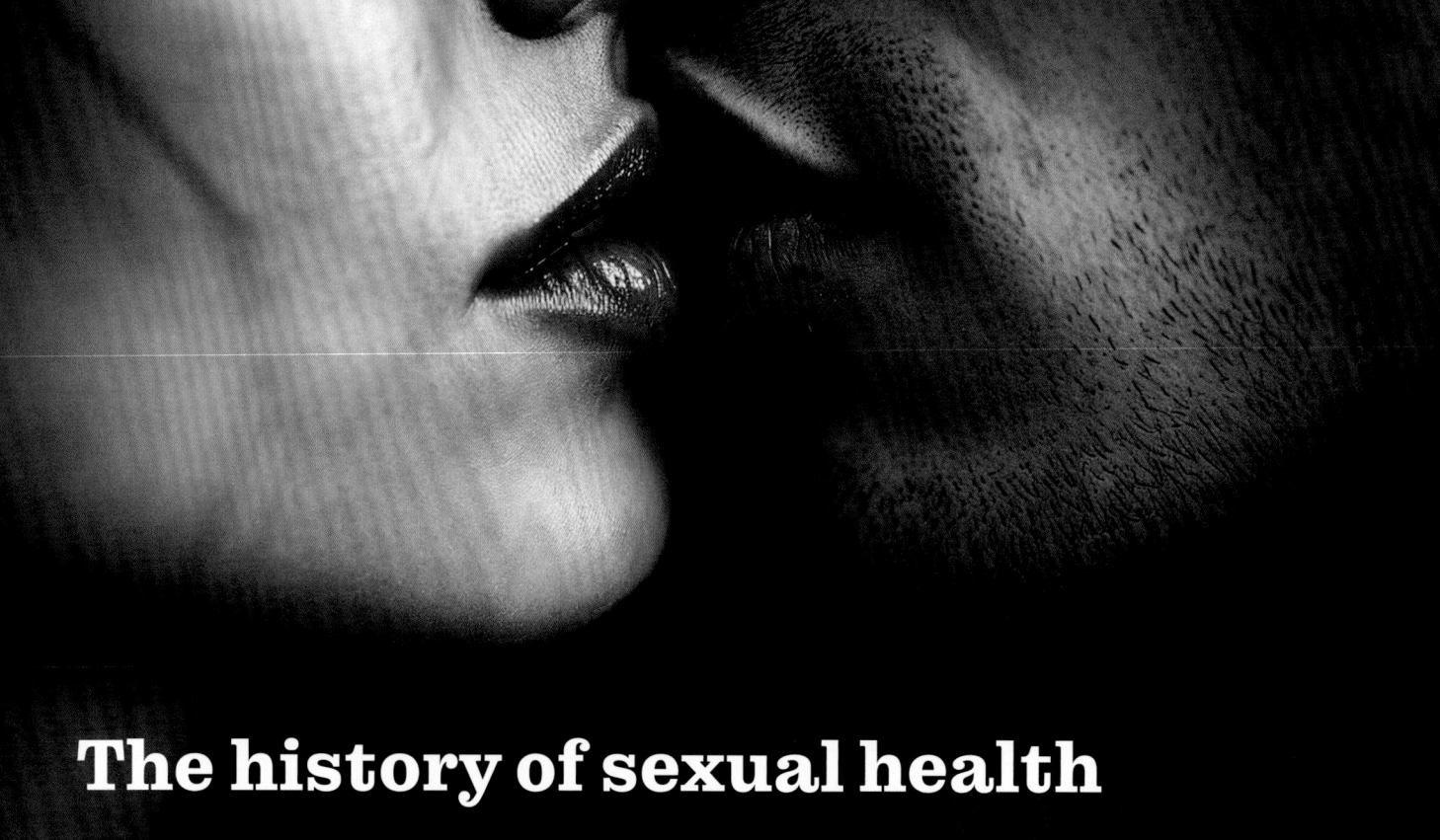

The history of sexual health

The World Health Organisation (WHO) defines sexual health as 'a state of physical, mental and social wellbeing in relation to sexuality'. It is an important area of public health and the current investment in England in sexual, reproductive and HIV services by local councils is around £534 million – the third largest area of public health spend. In England in 2021, over four million consultations at sexual health services (SHS) took place, nearly 16% more than the previous year.

Birth control

The modern birth control movement started in the late 19th century. A threat to the male dominated society, controlling fertility was believed to encourage infidelity and faced considerable opposition from the church, state and medical professionals. For example, when prominent atheists, Annie Besant and Charles Bradlaugh, re-published Charles Knowlton's *Fruits of Philosophy* – a leaflet which argued that it was 'more moral to prevent conception of children, than, after they are born, to murder them by want of food, air and clothing', they were charged and found guilty of breaching the Obscene Publications Act of 1857.

As is still the case, health outcomes were hugely dependent on women's circumstances and those who suffered the greatest were more likely to live in poverty and overcrowded squalor, suffer more from ill-health and infant mortality, and had no access to birth control.

During the early 20th century, the consensus between doctors remained that birth control led to prostitution and immorality, and the topic was not taught to medical students. In London in 1921, Marie Stopes, a biologist and campaigner, opened the first sexual health clinic in Britain, the Mothers' Clinic for Constructive Birth Control. The clinic was run by nurses rather than doctors, and female doctors were used for referrals. It was the first time qualified clinical staff gave contraceptive advice and it marked the beginning of Sexual Health Services (SHS) being a medical speciality rather than a social or commercial activity. Four years later, in May 1925, the first centre outside of London, in Wolverhampton, was opened.

Clinic numbers began to increase and in 1930, the National Birth Control Council (NBCC) was formed from 20 clinics so 'married people may space or limit their families and thus mitigate the evils of ill-health and poverty'.[ii] The NBCC coordinated the work of Maternity and Child Welfare Councils but, as had been true for decades, unmarried and working-class women were offered little support or opportunities to seek advice. By 1939, NBCC member societies merged into The Family Planning Association (FPA).

Following the NHS' formation in 1948, local authorities took over maternity and child welfare centres, providing discretionary provision of contraceptive advice. The FPA continued to campaign for the NHS to provide family planning services and in 1952 FPA clinics began to offer pre-marital advice to women.

During the 1960s, huge progress was made. The first oral contraceptive was introduced in 1961 and in 1967 laws surrounding sexuality began to change, accurately reflecting public attitudes and the problems faced by people in everyday society. The Abortion Act legalised abortion, in certain circumstances, in the UK and was a key public health driver, reducing the incidence of maternal mortality and morbidity. The Family Planning Act 1967 enabled local authorities to give contraceptive advice and supplies under the NHS and included unmarried women, although it was at the discretion of the authority.

Teenage pregnancy

Between 1993 and 2020, the under-18 conception rate in England and Wales decreased by 69%, from 42 per 1,000 women to 13 per 1,000 women. Rising educational and employment aspirations, changing housing availability, improved access to contraception and developments in sexual and reproductive health education in schools have all been credited as drivers of this fall. This dramatic reduction serves as evidence of the successes of public health interventions and exemplifies the positive impact of preventative action on health outcomes.

Whilst much progress has been made, the under-18 conception rate remains much higher than that of comparable European countries. Targeted interventions for young women living in high risk or deprived areas, universal access to reproductive and sexual health advice and increased funding across the four nations to deliver these services should remain a priority to continue the trend of declining conception rates and to bring the UK in line with equivalent European countries.[vi]

Sexually transmitted infections (STIs)

During the first world war about 5% of British troops were infected with a sexually transmitted infection (STI) and over 400,000 British or allied men were admitted to hospital as a result of one to over five times the hospitalisation rate for trench foot. By the middle of the war, 50% of infertility in women was caused by gonorrhoea and 30% of children in blind schools were there as a result of syphilis. In 1916, the Local Government Board issued the Public Health Venereal Diseases Regulations based on recommendations by the Royal Commission on Venereal Diseases. These regulations led to the development of a nationwide network of clinics based in hospitals in heavily populated areas offering free confidential diagnosis and treatment for syphilis, gonorrhoea and chancroid.

Attitudes began to change and there was a greater need to manage venereal disease as well as a greater recognition of its effects. It was thought that educating civil and military populations against the dangers of venereal disease and the importance of sexual hygiene would improve case rates.

Today, SHS in the UK encompass a wide variety of services, including the provision of sexual health or GUM clinics. STI screening, for infections such as chlamydia, gonorrhoea, syphilis or HIV are all available, as well as genital examinations, cervical screenings and advice on pregnancy and contraceptives.

In the 1980's a new STI was discovered – human immunodeficiency virus (HIV), which can lead to the development of the disease acquired immunodeficiency syndrome (AIDs). The HIV/AIDs crisis was a global public health emergency which for years highly stigmatised homosexual relationships and according to the WHO, has killed over 40.1 million people. The first diagnoses of an AIDS related illness in the UK was in 1981, and a report of the gentleman's death was published by *The Lancet*. By 1985, 58 AIDS-related deaths had been recorded in Britain. As a response to growing infection rates and hospitalisations, a year later the UK Government launched the major public health information campaign 'AIDS: don't die of ignorance'. A leaflet about AIDS was delivered to every household in the UK alongside a television advert designed to get people to read the information leaflet. By 1996, a combination of antiretroviral drugs, known as triple combination threat therapy (HAART), became standard treatment for HIV infection. HAART maintains the patient's immune system function and prevents opportunistic infection, which is often the cause of death. Crucially, it also prevents the transmission of HIV if the HIV-positive patient maintains an undetectable viral load. The use of HAART has saved millions of lives, reducing AIDs-related deaths by between 60% and 80%, and is noted to be one of the greatest public health success stories globally.

Over time, the stigma surrounding STIs has lessened and in 2002, the National Chlamydia Screening Programme was established to 'prevent and control chlamydia through early detection and treatment of asymptomatic infection; reduce onward transmission to sexual partners; and prevent the consequences of untreated infection'.

As a result of the 2012 Health and Social Care Act, sexual, reproductive health and HIV commissioning arrangements were split between NHS England and local authorities. The English HIV & Sexual Health Commissioners' Group (EHSHCG) was set up in 2013, supported by ADPH and funded by Local Government Association (LGA), as a collaborative network to support commissioners and improve the delivery of local, integrated services through sector-led improvement. It is now hosted by ADPH and funded through LAPH subscriptions.

As well as improvements in screening and treatment, further developments in preventing STIs have continued to emerge. For example, PrEP, pre-exposure prophylaxis, is a drug taken by those at risk of contracting HIV but are not yet infected, reducing the risk of contracting the virus after exposure by 99%. Improving PrEP take up is, however, heavily reliant on public health services and the EHSHCG have facilitated projects to increase access to PrEP, such as their PrEP Commissioning Champions, facilitating collaborative commissioning by working with NHSE and the DHSC.

In 2022, over two million sexual health screens for STIs took place at SHS, an increase of 13.4% compared to 2021. Both gonorrhoea and syphilis returned to the high levels of pre-pandemic reporting, and gonorrhoea diagnoses were the highest reported annually since records began.[viii] This is evidence of the continued need for well-funded, accessible SHS alongside public health messaging which successfully raises awareness of the importance of testing and treatment.

SHS in the UK have taken centuries to develop into the inclusive and vital public health provision that they are in the present day. Medical developments have allowed STIs to be controlled, and the introduction of HAART and PrEP curtailed a public health crisis that killed millions globally. However, effective SHS require much more than medical interventions alone, and the continued funding of and equitable access to education and support is vital for good sexual health practice.

30 August 2023

The above information is reprinted with kind permission from the Association of Directors of Public Health (UK).
© 2024 Association of Directors of Public Health (UK)

www.adph.org.uk

Where can I get sexual health advice, now?

Forgotten your pill or had unprotected sex? Maybe you're worried about something? Here's what to do and where to go if you need help urgently.

Could I have a sexually transmitted infection (STI)?

If you have had unprotected sex (without a condom), there's a chance you could have caught a sexually transmitted infection (STI).

Arrange to get tested if you:

- haven't got symptoms, but are worried you might have an STI
- have symptoms, such as an unusual discharge
- feel something is wrong

If you're sexually active, either stop having sex or make sure you use a condom until you get your test results and know for sure whether or not you have an STI.

If you do have an STI, using a condom will help prevent passing it on. Your sexual partners should also get tested.

You can get free, confidential advice and treatment from your GP or specialist clinics in your area, including if you're under 16.

Hospitals often have sexual health clinics (also known as GUM clinics), which test for and treat STIs.

There are also lots of places that are set up especially for young people.

Most STIs can be easily treated, so don't be scared of having a test and finding you do have an STI.

I think I might be pregnant

The first thing to do is find out for certain by taking a pregnancy test. The sooner you do this, the better.

There are lots of places where you can have a free pregnancy test and get confidential advice, even if you're under 16.

These include:

- sexual health clinics (GUM clinics)
- contraception clinics (also called family planning clinics)
- some young people's services – call the national sexual health helpline on 0300 123 7123 for details (Monday to Friday, 9am to 8pm, and Saturday and Sunday, 11am to 4pm)
- Brook centres – for under-25s - visit the Brook website for details
- some GP surgeries

You can also buy a pregnancy test from pharmacies or some supermarkets, which you can do yourself at home.

I'm pregnant

If you're pregnant and it's unplanned, you'll need to decide if you want to continue with the pregnancy.

If you decide to have an abortion, the sooner this is done, the easier and safer it is.

But you might want to take time making your decision, which is why it's important to find out if you're pregnant as soon as possible.

Nobody needs to know you're pregnant until you're ready to tell them.

You can ask to see a female doctor if it would make you feel more comfortable.

If you decide to continue with the pregnancy, you should start your pregnancy (antenatal) care as soon as possible.

This includes health checks for you and your baby. Your GP can discuss this with you.

I've had sex without a condom

If you have had sex without a condom or the condom splits or comes off, there's a risk of both pregnancy and STIs.

The best thing to do is act quickly. The quicker you act, the sooner you can prevent a pregnancy or get tested for an STI.

Pregnancy

You can get pregnant if you have sex without a condom or the condom splits or comes off.

In this case, to avoid pregnancy you can either:

- take the emergency contraceptive pill, sometimes called the morning-after pill, up to 72 hours (3 days) or 120 hours (5 days) after having unprotected sex, depending on the type of pill
- have an intrauterine device (IUD), sometimes called a coil, fitted up to 120 hours (5 days) after having unprotected sex

However, try to take emergency contraception before 3 days, or have the coil fitted before 5 days. The sooner you take it, the more effective they will be.

Take a pregnancy test if your next period doesn't arrive when you expect it to.

If you're having sex, don't regularly rely on emergency contraception to stop you getting pregnant.

There are lots of contraceptive options you can choose from.

Talk to a nurse or doctor at a clinic or GP surgery about what type of contraception is right for you.

STIs

If you have sex without a condom or the condom splits or comes off, you're also at risk of getting an STI.

If this happens and you're worried you have caught an STI, you can get confidential help and advice in your local area, as well as free testing for STIs, at:

- sexual health clinics (GUM clinics)
- some community contraceptive clinics
- some GPs

Chlamydia

Chlamydia is one of the most common STIs in the UK.

It can be easily tested for and testing is free and confidential at a sexual health clinic or GP surgery.

You can also buy chlamydia testing kits to use at home, with free tests available online for 15- to 24-year-olds.

I've forgotten to take my pill

You may not be protected against pregnancy if you have forgotten to take your pill.

This depends on the type you're taking, how many doses you have missed already, and how many pills are left in the packet.

If you have trouble remembering to take a pill every day, you could consider using another method of contraception, such as the contraceptive implant, contraceptive injection or IUD.

This means you don't have to think about your contraception every day or every time you have sex.

You may need to use condoms for extra protection.

If you need further advice, speak to a doctor, nurse or pharmacist as soon as possible.

Will medication or being ill affect my pill?

If you take it correctly, at the right time on the right day, the contraceptive pill is 99% effective.

But certain things, such as being sick (vomiting), can stop it working properly.

Always read the leaflet inside the packet so you know what might affect it.

Some medicines can prevent the pill working properly. Always ask your doctor or pharmacist to advise you about this if they're giving you any medicines.

I've been pushed into sex

If someone has forced or persuaded you into a sexual situation you're uncomfortable with, help is available.

You can call the national sexual health helpline free on 0300 123 7123, Monday to Friday, 9am to 8pm, Saturday and Sunday, 11am to 4pm. Your call will be treated with sensitivity and in strict confidence.

You can also contact a sexual assault referral centre (SARC), where you can get specialist support and medical care if you have been sexually assaulted.

A sexual assault can happen anywhere, including in your home, and is more likely to be carried out by someone you know rather than a stranger.

You can also ask at your GP surgery, contraceptive clinic or sexual health clinic.

If I use a sexual health service will they tell my parents?

Find out about confidential sexual health services, including contraception, testing for sexually transmitted infections (STIs) and advice on unplanned pregnancy, even if you're under 16 years old.

Sexual health services (contraception and pregnancy advice, or tests for STIs, including HIV) are free and confidential.

If you're 13 to 16, you have the same rights to confidentiality as an adult. The doctor, nurse or pharmacist will not tell your parents, or anyone else, as long as they believe that you fully understand the information and decisions involved.

They'll encourage you to consider telling your parents or carers, but they will not make you.

Even if the doctor, nurse or pharmacist feels that you're not mature enough to make a decision yourself, the consultation will still be confidential. They will not tell anyone that you saw them, or anything about what you said.

The only time a professional might want to tell someone else is if they believe there is a risk to your safety or welfare, such as abuse. The risk would need to be serious, and they would usually discuss this with you first.

The situation is different for people under 13, because the law says that people of this age cannot consent (say yes) to sexual activity. If you're under 13, doctors, nurses and health workers might feel it's in your best interests to involve other people, such as a social worker.

What you can get from sexual health services

If the healthcare worker feels that you understand the information and can make your own decision, you can get advice on the following:

- Contraception
- Emergency contraception (the morning-after pill or an intrauterine device [IUD])
- Condoms
- Unplanned pregnancy
- Tests and treatments for sexually transmitted infections (STIs), including HIV.

The above information is reprinted with kind permission from the NHS.
© Crown Copyright 2024
This information is licensed under the Open Government Licence v3.0
To view this licence, visit http://www.nationalarchives.gov.uk/doc/open-government-licence/

www.nhs.uk

What happens at a sexual health check-up?

An expert explains why STI testing is so important – for everyone.

By Katie Wright

With record levels of gonorrhoea and syphilis cases reported by the UK Health Security Agency, it's important to take sexual health seriously – and not just for young people.

In fact, the number of common sexually transmitted infections (STIs) among over-65s increased by 20% from 2017 to 2019, according to the Local Government Association.

This is why if you are sexually active, regular testing is necessary whatever your age – even if you don't have any symptoms.

'Sexual health check-ups are important because STIs can be silent but can also have significant health implications,' says Dr Priyanka Patel, consultant ambulatory gynaecologist at London Gynaecology.

'STIs such as chlamydia can affect female fertility, and STIs such as HIV weaken the immune system.'

To mark Sexual Health Week (September 11–17), Dr Patel talks through some key points about STI screening…

How often should you have an STI check?

'You need to have an STI check whenever you have a new partner, especially if you're not using condoms, or think you were exposed to an STI,' says Patel.

'Everyone should have an STI screen, including an HIV test, every year if having sex without condoms with new or casual partners.'

Testing is also advised for anyone who develops possible symptoms. These may include unusual discharge from the vagina, penis or anus; pain when peeing; blisters, sores, lumps or skin growths on the genitals or anus; itching or a rash.

What will you be asked at a check-up?

You can find your nearest sexual health clinic via the NHS to book an appointment. Many sexual health services now offer free self-sampling kits to order online for people who don't have any symptoms and want to do a check-up at home.

'Men may have to hold their urine before testing, but women do not need to do anything in particular to prepare,' Patel says.

'You will be asked about your sexual history, partners, contraceptive use and general health. You will be asked for details about your recent sexual partners and types of sex you have.'

These questions may feel personal or intrusive but are important to ensure the correct tests are done. Remember, taking care of your sexual health is about being safe and empowered and healthcare professionals are there to help.

What tests are done?

'The testing will depend on the answers you give about the types of sex you have,' says Patel. 'Vaginal, throat and anal swabs may be done – these will be used to test for chlamydia and gonorrhoea.'

To do this, the clinician rubs a cotton bud inside the area for a few seconds. A blood sample will be taken to test for syphilis and HIV.

Patel continues: 'If you have symptoms, then the clinician will usually carry out a speculum examination to look at the health of the vagina and cervix.'

How do you get STI test results?

The way your results are delivered varies between clinics, and they will advise when you should expect to hear back.

'Most will send results via a text message or give you a number to call for results,' says Patel, while some have a 'no news is good news' policy, meaning if you don't hear anything then you've got the all-clear.

For home testing kits, you'll get a notification to say your samples were received and results are usually sent via text message.

'If you test positive for an STI, they will arrange for treatment and offer support,' Patel explains – which goes for both clinic and self-sampling.

She adds: 'It's important to notify partners of any positive results and the sexual health clinic can also assist in anonymous partner notification.'

11 September 2023

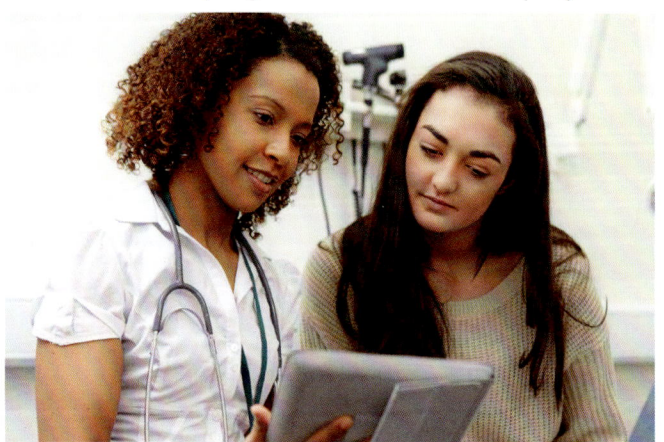

The above information is reprinted with kind permission from *The Independent*.

© independent.co.uk 2024

www.independent.co.uk

A comprehensive guide to smear tests

Screening for cervical cancer plays a crucial role in women's lives, contributing to cervical cancer prevention. Distinguished consultant in sexual and reproductive health Dr Emily Lord explains everything you need to know about smear tests, answering your frequently asked questions about the programme.

What is a smear test?

The cervical cancer screening programme plays a pivotal role in women's healthcare. 'Having your smear test' taken involves a speculum examination, where a small plastic device is inserted into the vagina to visualise the cervix. A brush sample is taken, sent to a special lab to check for any evidence of human papillomavirus (HPV). Detecting HPV early allows for timely treatment, often preventing cancer development.

What is HPV?

HPV is a group of sexually transmitted viruses, highly prevalent with over 70% of sexually active individuals experiencing infection, most people clear the virus on their own within months. There are over 200 strains; while some types of HPV cause harmless skin warts, other 'high-risk' strains may cause changes in the cells. Persistent high-risk HPV types can lead to cervical cancer (and cancers within the oropharynx and anogenital regions). Over 99% of cervical cancer cases are caused by persistent HPV infection, (Okunade 2020).

HPV types affecting the genitals can be classified into high-risk (oncogenic) and low-risk (non-oncogenic) categories, based on their association with the development of cervical cancer and its early-stage lesions.

Low-risk types: 6, 11, 42, 43, and 44

High-risk types: 16, 18, 31, 33, 35, 39, 45, 51, 52, 56, 58, 59, 68, 73, and 82. Types 16 and 18, account for 70% of cervical cancer cases.

The UK smear programme

Cisgender women and trans-males aged 25 to 64 are invited for smear tests regularly. Testing frequency varies by age: every 3 years for ages 25 to 49, and every 5 years for ages 50 to 64. Samples are initially tested for high-risk HPV, with cytology performed if detected. Treatment involves a colposcopy examination, where the clinician can look closely at the cervix using a special microscope (which stays outside of your body). If needed, a small biopsy may be taken to further assess areas that look abnormal.

Frequently asked questions

I am a virgin – do I need a smear?

If somebody has never had any form of sex or sexual contact – their risk of developing cervical cancer is very low. However, 'low risk' is not 'no risk'. HPV can also be passed on from oral sex, genital touching or sharing sex toys. Talk to your clinician to discuss the best option for you.

I suffer from vulval pain and really struggle with a speculum, what can be done to help me with my smear?

Having a speculum and a smear can be uncomfortable, but if you suffer from vulval pain already (including vaginismus and vulvodynia) it can be especially challenging and may mean you delay having it done. It is important you discuss your worries with your doctor, there are lots of things that can be done to help the process, for example ensuring your clinician uses a small speculum, a small amount of lubrication, or even sometimes a little bit of local anaesthetic gel. They key is helping you be as relaxed as possible, taking time and ensuring you feel in control of the procedure.

I do not identify as female, but have a cervix – do I need a smear?

Trans men and non-binary people assigned female at birth still need to have their smear test taken. A few important things to note – if you have changed your gender with your GP, then you will not get your automatic invite (which only goes out to individuals registered as female) – so speak to your GP surgery to ensure that you are still on the recall. Also, if you are taking testosterone, you may have vaginal dryness and this may make the process a little more uncomfortable – speak to your clinician before the test to ensure they do everything possible to make it as easy as possible.

Do I need to go for a smear test if I've had the HPV vaccine?

Yes. The vaccine does not protect you from all types of HPV, so it is important to still go for your smear when you are called.

Can I still go for a cervical screening if I'm pregnant?

It is best to not have your smear when you are pregnant, as it can make the results harder to interpret. If you are planning a pregnancy, make sure you have your smear, (if it is due) before you conceive.

Can you get tested for all the HPV types?

On the NHS programme, they test for the most common types of high-risk HPV (16,18). This is because they are the most likely to cause cervical cancer. It is possible to have a private smear test taken, which can assess for all high risk (and low risk) HPV subtypes. You should discuss this option with your clinician.

8 March 2024

The above information is reprinted with kind permission from Top Doctors.
© 2024 Top Doctors

www.topdoctors.co.uk

Genital hygiene

The genital area, including the surrounding skin, is very delicate and can easily be damaged. There are a number of ways to protect and look after your genital skin.

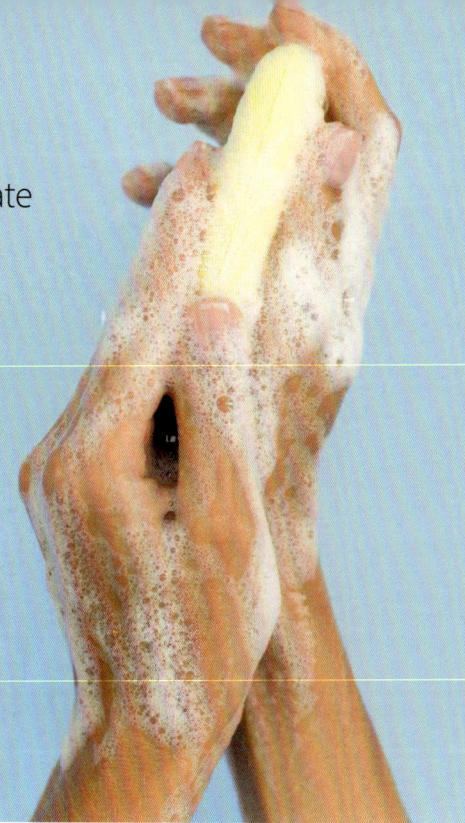

By Abbey Eboigbe – Senior Nurse – HIV and Sexual Health

Don't

- Don't use soaps or shower gel, including feminine hygiene products, to cleanse your genitals. These products are often the leading cause of genital dryness, itching and irritation. Even those that claim to be 'mild' or 'unperfumed' can cause irritation; it is the foaming agent (lauryl sulphate) that people are sensitive to.

- Don't over wash! Washing your genitals once a day is adequate. If you over wash, you will wash away your good, healthy bacteria. Doing this means 'bad' bacteria may colonise and cause you symptoms.

- Don't douche! Douching, like over washing, runs the risk of washing away those healthy bacteria. This can again lead to soreness, dryness and irritation. It can even cause damage to the delicate lining of the vagina or anus, leaving you more susceptible to infections, including HIV.

- Don't remove pubic hair! Pubic hair is there for a reason! It protects our genitals from external irritants, such as dirt and bacteria – much like the role of the hair on our heads, our eyelashes and eyebrows. Shaving and hair removal products cause damage to sensitive genital skin, causing irritation and localised infection such as folliculitis. It can also leave us more prone to outbreaks of genital warts and herpes simplex virus (HSV). Our skin is our first defence and if it is inflamed or broken, it provides a portal of entry, allowing these viruses to spread around the area.

- Don't use sanitary wear unnecessarily! Sanitary towels and tampons are designed to collect blood loss (menses) during your period only. Wearing these at other times prevents our skin from being able to breathe. It can cause excess heat and sweating to the area, resulting in soreness, itching and irritation. If you have a vaginal secretion, which is perfectly normal, then it is better to change your underwear more frequently.

Do

- Do use plain water or an emollient to wash your genitals. Whilst water is fine to use alone, we recommend washing with an emollient such as aqueous cream, diprobase or double base. These are available from a pharmacy or supermarket (and online) and are very cost effective. You can apply the emollient like a cream to your genital skin before getting in the bath or shower, this will act like a barrier to other soaps and shampoos you might use. Rinse the area well when you are finished washing. Emollients are safe for daily use. If you have dry genital skin apply some before bed every night.

- Do allow fresh air to get to your genital skin! During the winter months, our genitals rarely get a chance to breathe due to us wearing multiple layers to keep warm! And in the summer, our genitals can get hot and sweaty, due to the temperature outside! When you can, e.g., when you're at home in the evening watching TV and when you are sleeping – try to go underwear free! A loose-fitting pair of pyjama bottoms works well, to cover your modesty but allows some air flow to get to the area.

- Do wear cotton (or cotton gusset) underwear. Cotton material allows our skin to breathe, whereas manmade fibres don't and can make your skin hot, causing irritation. You should preferably use a non-biological washing powder/liquid to wash your underwear.

Frequently asked questions about genital hygiene: our tips

I think I might have thrush or BV, what do I do?

The symptoms of conditions like thrush and BV can often be easily managed using the genital hygiene advice on this page, and most episodes will clear with this alone. Over the counter treatments for thrush and BV may also help, these can be bought in a pharmacy or supermarket.

I have tried the advice on this page, but I am still itching and sore, what do I do?

If you have followed the advice on this page and you continue to have symptoms, it would be important for you to contact the clinic for further advice and assessment.

Symptoms of itching, irritation and dryness can take sometime to resolve, so it is important that you allow a bit of time for this to happen.

I have been having tummy pain and an unusual discharge, what should I do?

If your symptoms include abdominal pain (especially during or after sex), unexpected bleeding or an offensive discharge, then you must contact your clinic for a consultation without delay. These symptoms can be an indicator of something more serious going on and require an examination, and tests to be done.

I don't have dry or irritated skin, can I continue using shower gel to wash?

In short – yes! you can.

However, we would still recommend switching to water only or an emollient, as using these can prevent itching, irritation and dryness from happening. Think of it as your skin care routine for your genitals!

I have read this advice, thanks! I don't have any symptoms – do I need to worry?

You don't need to worry, but it is important to know that most sexually transmitted infections (STI's) come without symptoms. If you are sexually active then it is important to test for STI's. We recommend testing at the beginning AND end of a relationship. If you are having casual partners, then testing at least once a year is ideal.

Getting a check-up is easy, you can call a sexual health clinic, or if you are under 25 you can order a home testing kit.

Our top 5 tips for healthy bits!

The genital area, including the surrounding skin is very delicate and can easily be damaged. Here are our top 5 tips for healthy genitals!

- Avoid irritants! Using soap, shower gel and feminine hygiene products can cause dryness, itching and irritation. Wash with plain water or an emollient instead!

- Don't overwash! Washing once a day is enough! You run the risk of washing away good, healthy bacteria's by washing too much, and douching is a no-no!

- Do allow your genitals some fresh air! – and this doesn't have to mean walking around half naked! Sleeping underwear free allows air to circulate to the part of your body that is covered up the most! Wearing breathable cotton (or cotton gusset) undies is advised too, and you should wash these in non-bio!

- Don't remove your pubic hair! Whilst it might be fashionable to have a Brazilian or Hollywood, pubic hair serves a purpose. It stops bacteria and dirt from getting into our genitals and causing problems!

- Do get regular sexual health check-up's to make sure you are free from infection. Most STIs don't come with symptoms, so testing for them is important. We suggest, at the beginning AND end of a relationship, or at least once a year if you are having casual partners.

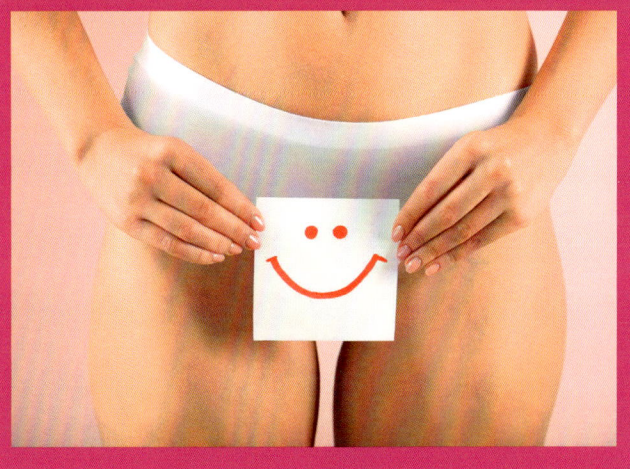

The above information is reprinted with kind permission from Royal Devon University Healthcare NHS Foundation Trust.

© 2024 Royal Devon University Healthcare NHS Foundation Trust

www.devonsexualhealth.nhs.uk

Consent

When it comes to sex or any kind of intimate activity with a partner, whether you're in a relationship with them or not, consent is key.

Consent is about your choice when it comes to having sex with someone. It's also about saying what you are and aren't comfortable with doing when it comes to sex – whether it's kissing, touching or anything else.

What is consent?

Consent is when you want something to happen and agree to it. It's important that no one ever does anything sexual to you unless you consent – it's your body and no one should ever do anything to you that you don't want.

If someone puts pressure on you by saying things like 'Come on, you won't know if you like it until you try', uses threats to try to get you to do things by saying things like 'You wouldn't want me to post that picture on Snapchat/Instagram would you?' or tries to manipulate you by saying things like 'I thought you were cool/more experienced', they're not respecting you and it wouldn't be consent.

It doesn't matter if you've done something with that person before, even if you're in a relationship with them, they're your ex or someone you're friends with – it's about whether you wanted to do it then, in that moment. And even if you've started having sex or being intimate with each other and then changed your mind, you can stop or decide you don't like it any more, at any time.

Is it just about saying no?

Consent can be verbal and non-verbal.

You don't have to say the word 'no' to someone to imply you don't or no longer consent to sexual activity.

If a partner tries pushing you away, or freezes, or doesn't seem comfortable with what is happening – stop and ask if they are okay. Ask if they want to continue. And respect whatever decision they make.

'They did say no but they seem like they want to – should I just make them have sex anyway?'

No means no. If someone does say they don't want to have sex or do anything with you, you should respect their decision.

'They were flirting with me/They were wearing a revealing outfit – they must want to have sex…'

Flirting is not an invitation to sex. Wearing a revealing outfit is not 'asking for it'.

The only way to know if someone wants to have sex with you is to ask and get their consent to do so.

Even if you're already engaged in sexual activity with someone, either of you can change your mind at any time, and it's important to stop the activity and respect this decision if your partner does this.

'My partner has had sex before/We've had sex before, so they must be okay with it?'

It doesn't matter if someone has had sex before or hasn't, even if it is with you.

You still need to ask if they want to have sex and talk about what you are both comfortable doing. Maybe they are okay

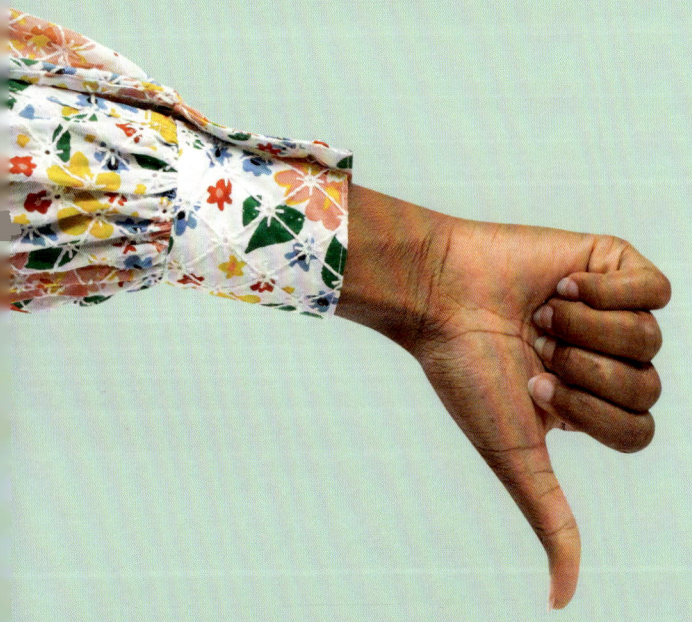
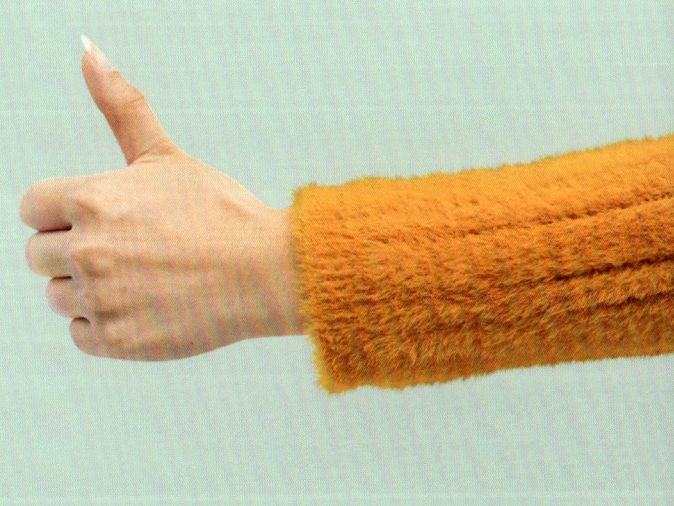

with kissing but not touching. Maybe they want to have sex but don't want to do certain things. You need to talk about this.

You need to have consent every time. It doesn't matter if you've never had sex before or had sex together multiple times – you need to make sure your partner consents and is okay with everything. Just because they've done something before doesn't mean they are okay with it every time.

'They want to have sex but I don't, should I do it anyway?'

You should never feel pressured to have sex or engage in any kind of sexual activity that you are not comfortable with.

Sex should be an activity that you both enjoy and get pleasure from. If you don't want to have sex, then you shouldn't force yourself to do so just because someone else wants to, and they should respect you and your decision.

At what age can you consent to sex?

It's important that people are ready before they start having sexual relationships (eg. any kind of sexual activity) with others. This is so you understand enough about sex and how you feel about it, what you like and what you don't like. And so you're old enough to understand and respect how the other person feels too.

The law says you can consent to most kinds of sexual activity from age 16.

If you're aged 12 or under, the law says it's not possible for you to consent to any kind of sexual activity, and so no one is allowed to have sex with you or touch you in a sexual way. This is to protect you. It would never be your fault if someone did this to you – even if you agreed to it or went along with it.

If you're aged 13, 14 or 15, the law says that no one aged 16 or above is allowed to have sex with you or touch you in a sexual way, even if you consent.

If both people are aged 13, 14, or 15, the law says they're not allowed to have sexual intercourse with each other (where the penis goes inside the vagina, mouth or anus) or oral sex (where the mouth touches the vagina, anus or penis) even if you both consent.

Young people aged 13, 14 or 15 can lawfully consent to other things like touching and kissing with each other. But it's really important that there's no pressure – it's only consent if you feel ready and freely choose to do something, without being pressured.

Consent, alcohol and drugs

The law says that you're not able to give consent if you are incapable because of the influence of alcohol and/or drugs. So no one should initiate having sex with you if you're too drunk or influenced by drugs because you're not able to make a clear decision about what you want to do.

How drunk is too drunk?

This will be different for everyone – it's not about how many units, because alcohol affects everyone differently. The point is that no one should try to have sex with you if they're not sure that you're thinking clearly and you're in control of your decisions. For example – if you don't seem as in control as you usually are, if your speech is a bit slurred, if you're not walking straight, if you're feeling dizzy or sick, if you're not fully conscious… all of these things indicate you're probably (or definitely in some cases) not able to make clear decisions about what you want to do, and other people should respect this.

What if we were both drunk?

Even if both people were drinking (or using drugs), sexual intercourse doesn't just 'happen' – someone has to get things started or take things further. And if they are affected by alcohol, they are still responsible for their actions if they have sex with someone who can't consent.

I'm worried people might say I 'put myself at risk' if I drank alcohol

It is never your fault or your responsibility if someone has sex with you when you're not able to consent or you didn't want to have sex with them.

There are lots of good reasons for being careful about alcohol and drugs – like your health and mental wellbeing, and the law. But responsibility for rape always lies with the perpetrator (the person who did it) and never the person they assaulted.

What about consent for young people with learning disabilities?

The law says that to be able to consent to sexual activity, a person with a learning disability needs to:

- be old enough (for example over 16 for sexual intercourse),
- understand what sexual activity they might do involves,
- be able to make decisions about what they want to do and don't want to do, and
- be able to communicate their decisions.

17 May 2024

The above information is reprinted with kind permission from Young Scot.
© 2024 Young Scot

www.young.scot

When is someone mentally ready to have sex?

Here are three essential questions to determine if you are ready for sex.

By David W. Wahl Ph.D.

Of the many questions I am asked every day about sex, one that has recently been common is: 'When can I tell that I am ready to have sex?' Those asking the question are not talking about being physically ready, they are asking about mental readiness. Are they psychologically ready? Are they emotionally ready? One may think that those who are asking me this question are most likely young – teenagers. Well, yes, teenagers do ask me this question, but I also have adults that ask the same question.

When is someone in the right frame of mind to begin having sex? There is certainly not a one-size-fits-all answer to this question. Becoming sexually active is a major event in an individual's life and we all respond to it differently. As with any new turning point in the life course, the psychological reaction is unique to the individual. So, there is not a set answer to the question of sexual readiness. However, I can offer questions each person should contemplate before becoming sexually active. Your own personal readiness should be evident to you through your responses. The questions centre around three primary topics to consider: communication, maturity, and responsibility.

Communication: I have long argued that open and transparent communication is the most important aspect of a healthy sexual relationship. I believe this to be true even if the sexual activity is not part of an ongoing relationship. Communication is equally important in a one-night stand. The question you must ask yourself is whether you are able to talk to your partner about sex in an open manner. Can you tell them what you desire? Can you discuss your boundaries? Are you willing to discuss your expectations? Are you able to listen to what they have to say in a non-judgemental way? Are you willing to help create an environment wherein transparent dialogues about sex are valued? Are you able to communicate your concerns? If you answer 'no' to any of these questions, you will want to look more closely at why. You may come to the conclusion that you might not be ready yet to start a sexual relationship.

Maturity: This relates to how you will respond to both positive and negative reactions from your partner. This also includes how open you are to expressing your reactions to a partner. Are you able to let your partner know if you are uncomfortable with anything? Things may occur, both physically and emotionally, that you did not expect. How do you respond to uncertainty? How well are you able to react to the unexpected? You also have to recognise whether this is something that you want to do, instead of being pressured into having sex (consent is everything). Can you set boundaries and respect your partner's boundaries? Are you comfortable with yourself and your body? Are you able to trust your partner? Sex lives are not static. Things will change as time goes on. Can you respond to changes along the way in a mature manner?

Responsibility: Closely connected to maturity, one has to consider whether they are responsible enough to accept and deal with all possible outcomes from a sexual relationship. For instance, even if you properly communicate and negotiate the use of contraceptives, there is no contraceptive that is 100% effective, apart from abstinence. If the contraceptive fails, what is your responsibility? Are you responsible and mature enough to handle the situation in a sound and effective manner? Can you be counted on to be responsible for any possible outcome that results from sexual activity? Do you believe your partner would be equally responsible?

Surrounding these topics, a healthy education in matters of all things sexual is essential. Too many people enter into sexual relationships misinformed and lacking sexual education. Overall, an emphasis must be placed on the maintenance of sexual health, which the World Health Organization defines as '...a state of physical, emotional, mental and social wellbeing in relation to sexuality; it is not merely the absence of disease, dysfunction or infirmity. Sexual health requires a positive and respectful approach to sexuality and sexual relationships, as well as the possibility of having pleasurable and safe sexual experiences, free of coercion, discrimination and violence. For sexual health to be attained and maintained, the sexual rights of all persons must be respected, protected and fulfilled.' Just as many people enter into sexual relationships misinformed, they also engage in sexual relationships that are not compatible with sexual health.

While I, and others, can aid in guiding you to a conclusion about sexual readiness, the ultimate decision on whether you are ready for sexual activity is completely in your court. There are many questions you need to reflect on before that final decision is made. If you can openly communicate with your partner, keep yourself sexually educated, and if you have reflected on and believe you can sustain a high standard of maturity and responsibility, then I would have to say you are off to a good start.

14 July 2023

The above information is reprinted with kind permission from *Psychology Today*.
© 2024 Sussex Publishers, LLC

www.psychologytoday.com

How do I know if I am ready to have sex?

Figuring out if you're ready to have sex is a big decision, and it's not one to take lightly. You might feel pressure from friends, social media, or even movies and TV shows, where it seems like everyone is doing it and acting confident about it. But the truth is, not everyone is having sex, and even if they are, it doesn't mean you need to rush into it. What's important is that you feel ready, and that decision is entirely up to you.

If you're thinking about having sex for the first time or getting intimate with a new partner, it's important to take a step back and think carefully. Below are seven key things to consider before deciding if you're truly ready:

1. Your choice, your power

Remember this: your body, your rules. Just because someone else is ready doesn't mean you have to be. You should never feel pressured to say yes to sex, whether it's from friends, your partner, or society. If you're not sure or don't feel ready, it's totally okay to say no. 'No' is a complete sentence, and you don't need to justify your decision to anyone.

2. Respect the 'no'

On the flip side, it's just as important to respect your partner's decision if they say no or don't seem ready. Pushing someone to do something they don't want to is never okay. Consent is the foundation of any healthy relationship, and if both people aren't fully on board, then it's not the right time.

3. Know the deal with the law

In the UK, the legal age of consent is 16. This means that it's against the law to have sex with someone under that age. However, just because you're legally allowed to have sex at 16 doesn't mean you're automatically ready. Emotional readiness is just as important as physical readiness. It's essential to understand that age is only one part of the equation, and you should never feel pressured by the law or social norms to make this decision.

4. Consent is key

Consent is more than just saying 'yes'. It's about giving enthusiastic, ongoing permission to engage in sexual activity. If someone is drunk, high, or otherwise impaired, they can't legally or ethically give consent. Engaging in sex without consent is considered rape. Both you and your partner need to be fully present and aware when deciding to have sex.

5. Talk it out with your partner

Good communication with your partner is crucial before having sex. Discuss what you both feel comfortable with,

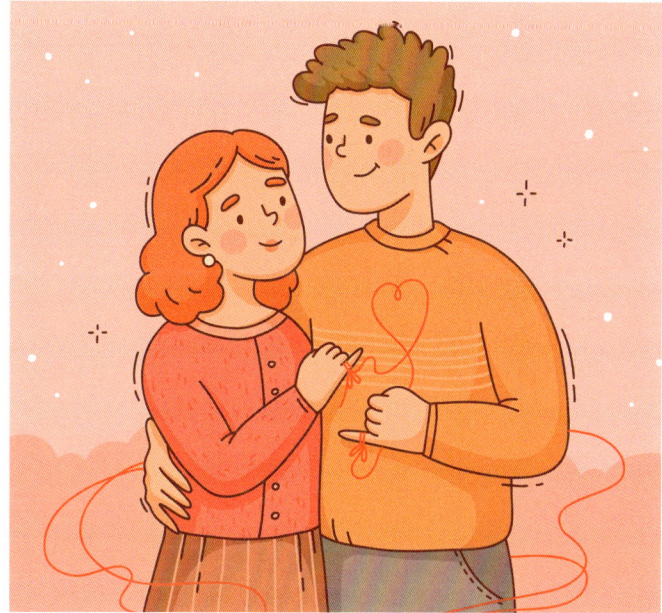

your boundaries, and your expectations. If you can't talk openly about sex, it's a sign that maybe you're not ready to take that step yet. Being able to communicate is a huge part of a healthy relationship, especially when it comes to something as personal as sex.

6. Safety first

Talking about protection is non-negotiable. Sex should always involve a conversation about using condoms or other forms of birth control to protect against sexually transmitted infections (STIs) and unwanted pregnancies. Even if it feels awkward, it's way more important to stay safe than to avoid an uncomfortable conversation. Always have a plan in place for protection before getting intimate.

7. You might not be ready to have sex if...

If just thinking about talking to your partner about sex makes you nervous or uncomfortable, that's a sign you might not be ready. And guess what? That's completely fine! There's no rush, no deadline, and no right or wrong time to have sex. It's a personal decision, and feeling 100% sure is key to avoiding regrets.

At the end of the day, navigating your sexual journey is a personal experience. There's no need to rush, no pressure to fit in, and definitely no shame in waiting until you feel completely ready. Everyone's timeline is different, and that's okay. Take the time to think through your decision and always listen to your gut. The most important thing is that you make choices that feel right for you, and you never regret them.

Stay safe, stay informed, and most importantly, stay true to yourself!

10 mega myths about sex

There are lots of things said about sex that aren't really true.

1. Real-life sex is like pornography

Not true – People taking part in most pornography are paid actors and they're doing things to entertain the people watching it.

Often, the things that happen all the time in porn aren't really common in everyday sex, but watching lots of porn can make people believe they are.

The way porn stars look is often very different to real life too.

2. Everyone is having sex

Not true – The decision to have sex is not about what other people are doing. Having sex is a personal choice and just because you have done it before, doesn't mean you have to do it again.

If you don't feel ready, you're not ready. You may not feel ready until you meet someone you trust and are comfortable with, and it's the next step in your relationship at a time that's right for both of you.

3. Boys don't need to worry about contraception, that is the girl's responsibility

Not true – The decision to have sex is a joint one. You might believe your girlfriend is on the pill or taking other contraception, but this is only effective if taken correctly.

Also, the only way to protect against a sexually transmitted infection (STI) is by using a condom.

4. STI tests are only for those who sleep around

Not true – Anyone who has unprotected oral, vaginal and anal sex can catch an STI, so it's always best to practice safe sex.

It's not always possible to tell if someone has an STI, and they might not even realise themselves if they don't have any symptoms.

Yearly tests are recommended, or each time you want to sleep with a different partner.

5. You can't get pregnant if you have sex in a bath, standing up and on your first time

Not true – There are lots of myths around having sex, buts that's exactly what they are – myths!

If you have any unprotected sex at any time, you are at risk of getting pregnant.

6. I would be able to tell if my partner had a STI

Not true – There is no way of being certain that your partner doesn't have an STI unless you both have been tested.

Before you consider having sex, it's important to talk to your partner about a full STI screen to make sure you both know for certain.

Condoms are the best protection for you both against STIs.

7. You can't use condoms if you're allergic to latex

Not true – Condoms come in all different sizes and latex-free condoms are also available if you have a latex allergy.

If you struggle to use condoms, take time to practice putting them on so you feel more comfortable with using them.

8. If he 'pulls out' when he comes (ejaculates), she can't get pregnant

Not true – Before a boy ejaculates, there's sperm in the pre-ejaculatory fluid (sometimes called pre-come), which leaks out when he gets an erection.

It only takes one sperm to get a girl pregnant. If you have unprotected sex, you're at risk of pregnancy and of catching an STI.

9. Drinking alcohol or using drugs aren't good when it comes to sex

True – When you're drunk or under the influence of drugs, it's hard to make smart decisions.

Alcohol and drugs can make you take risks, such as having sex before you're ready, or having sex with someone you don't trust.

You're more likely to regret having sex if you do it when you're drunk. You may also be at risk of a sexual assault and rape. If you're too drunk, you can't legally consent to sex.

10. You have to use emergency contraception the morning after sex

Not true – This is a common misconception due to the nickname for the emergency hormonal contraception pill being the 'morning-after pill'.

The emergency contraception pill can be given up to 5 days after unprotected sex, although the sooner it's taken the better.

If you're worried you have missed this time frame, there are other options available, so speak to your school nurse.

11 October 2023

The above information is reprinted with kind permission from the Health for Teens/NHS.

© Crown Copyright 2024

This information is licensed under the Open Government Licence v3.0
To view this licence, visit http://www.nationalarchives.gov.uk/doc/open-government-licence/

www.healthforteens.co.uk

Chapter 2: Contraception

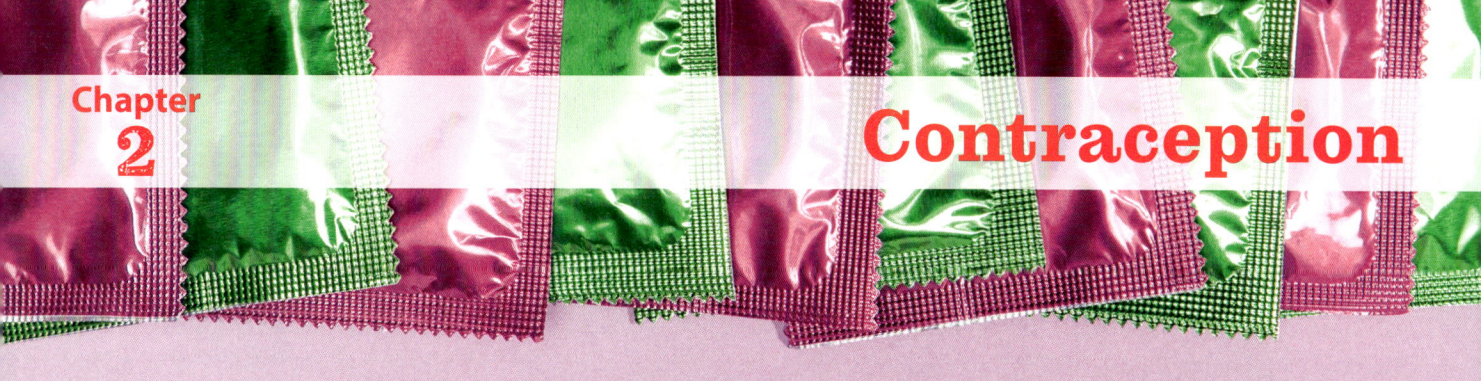

Why is contraception important?

Contraception, often referred to as birth control, is not just about avoiding unplanned pregnancies; it also plays a significant role in preventing sexually transmitted infections (STIs).

Empowering choices

One of the primary reasons contraception is essential is that it gives teenagers the power to make informed choices about their bodies and their futures. Deciding when to have children is a significant decision that impacts an individual's life trajectory. Access to contraception means you can plan your future without the added pressure of an unplanned pregnancy. This is crucial not just for females but for males too, as both partners share equal responsibility.

Relationship quality

Relationships during the teenage years are a crucial part of personal development. However, an unplanned pregnancy can put undue strain on these relationships, whether it's between the couple involved or with their respective families. Using contraception allows relationships to grow and mature naturally, without the added pressures and challenges an unplanned pregnancy might bring.

Preventing STIs

Aside from preventing unwanted pregnancies, certain forms of contraception, like condoms, play a pivotal role in preventing the spread of sexually transmitted infections (STIs). STIs can have serious health consequences, and in some cases, they can be life-threatening. Using barrier methods like condoms not only helps prevent pregnancy but also protects against STIs, making it a dual-purpose tool in sexual health.

Mental health considerations

Unplanned pregnancies can have a profound impact on a teenager's mental health. The stress, anxiety, and societal pressure can lead to depression and other mental health issues. Having access to and using contraception can alleviate these concerns, providing peace of mind and contributing to better overall mental health.

Equality and responsibility

Contraception is not just a female issue; it's equally important for males. It promotes equality by ensuring that both partners share the responsibility of preventing unwanted pregnancies and protecting against STIs. This shared responsibility can also enhance communication and trust within a relationship, laying a solid foundation for mutual respect and understanding.

Types of contraception

Understanding the different types of contraception available is key. These range from barrier methods (condoms and diaphragms) to hormonal (birth control pills, patches, injections) and natural methods (tracking fertility). Each type has its pros and cons, and what works best for one person may not be suitable for another. Therefore, consulting with a healthcare provider to find the most appropriate method is crucial.

Accessibility and education

Despite its importance, access to contraception and comprehensive education on how to use it effectively remains a challenge in many parts of the world. Advocating for accessible, affordable contraception and sexual education is essential. It empowers teenagers to make informed decisions about their sexual health, reducing the rates of unwanted pregnancies and STIs.

The bigger picture

Contraception is not just a personal choice or health issue; it affects the wellbeing of communities. By ensuring that teenagers have access to and understand how to use contraception, societies can reduce healthcare costs, increase educational and economic opportunities, and promote healthier and more prosperous communities.

Conclusion

Understanding the importance of contraception is vital for teenagers as they navigate their way into adulthood. It's not just about preventing unplanned pregnancies; it's about allowing young people the freedom to choose their paths without unnecessary obstacles. It's about safeguarding physical and mental health, ensuring brighter futures, and promoting responsibility and equality. As we move forward, let's continue the conversation about contraception, breaking down barriers and fostering an environment where informed choices lead to healthier lives for all.

Remember, it's okay to have questions and seek advice. Whether it's a healthcare provider, a trusted adult, or reliable resources, such as *Issues Online*, seeking out information is the first step in taking control of your sexual health and future. Don't shy away from these conversations; they're an important part of growing up and taking responsibility for your body and your choices.

Contraception and you

By Dr Dawn Harper

We have more contraceptive options today than ever before, but with choice can come confusion, so let's have a look at what is available.

I think of contraception in 5 categories:

1. Barrier methods
2. Hormonal methods – pills patches and rings
3. Long-acting reversible methods
4. Natural methods
5. Emergency contraception

Barrier methods

Male condoms

Condoms are often the first form of contraception used by a couple. They are most commonly made of latex, but some people are allergic to latex and thankfully you can get alternatives made of substances like silicone or polyurethane.

They come in different sizes and it is important you use the right size for you – too small and it might split, too big and it could come off, both of which runs the risk of an unwanted pregnancy. Most erect penises are between 5.5 and 6.5 inches and a standard fit condom is designed for this size.

To be used properly, the condom should be held in place and the penis removed from the vagina after ejaculation but before the penis becomes flaccid again to ensure that no semen enters the vagina.

Female condoms

The female condom is far less popular and is less effective than the male condom, but it does have the advantage that it can be inserted into the vagina anytime and doesn't require the penis to be erect first. It does take some getting used to though and you need to be confident that you can fit it properly so that it doesn't slip.

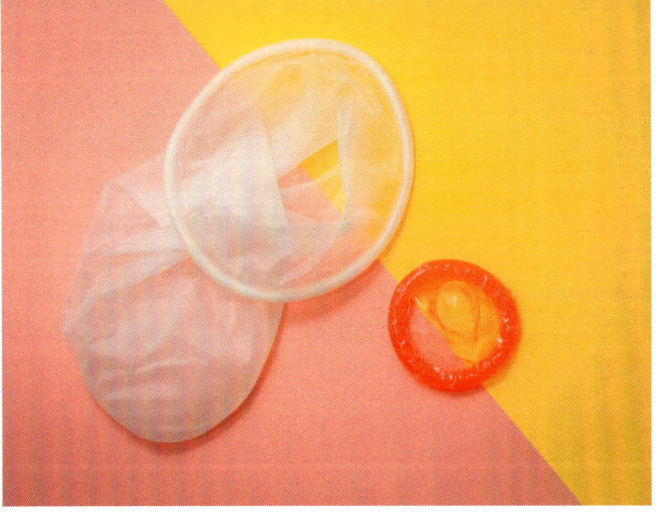

Diaphragms and caps

Diaphragms and caps are dome shaped and designed to fit over the cervix preventing sperm from getting into the womb. They are used with spermicide. They come in different sizes. If you choose this form of contraception you will need to see a GP or nurse at your GP surgery or a Family Planning Clinic so that they can advise on the best size for you and teach you how to fit it for yourself. To be used properly, a diaphragm or cap can be put in place anytime up to three hours before intercourse, but it must stay in place for at least six hours after sex.

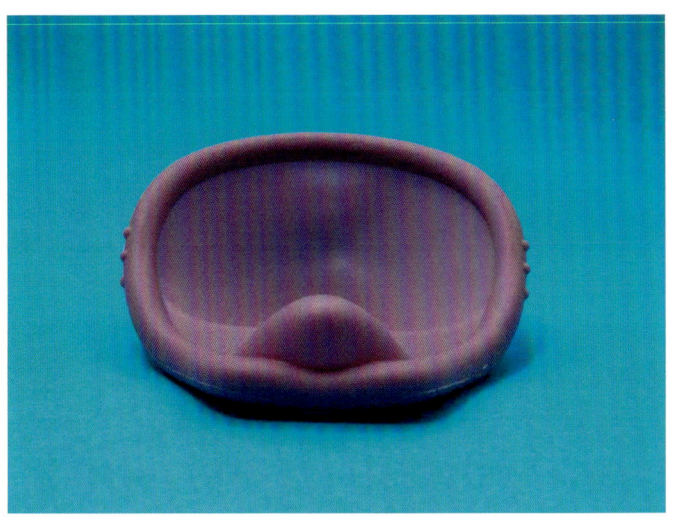

Hormonal methods

The Combined Oral Contraceptive Pill (COCP)

This is one of the most commonly used contraceptive methods – in fact it is thought that around one in four women use this method. As its name implies it is a combination pill containing two hormones – oestrogen and progestogen. It works by preventing ovulation, thickening cervical mucus and thinning the lining of the womb. It is the thinning that explains why many women find the bleeding they experience using the COCP is lighter than their normal period. It should be taken at the same time every day, but actually there is a 12-hour window, so if you miss a pill and remember within 12 hours you simply take the missed pill and then continue taking the rest of the packet at the same time each day. The COCP should be taken every day for three weeks and then you take a break for a week when you will experience a 'withdrawal bleed'. It is important that the next pack is started exactly a week later. Some brands of COCP contain 28 pills in a strip with the last seven pills in the pack being 'dummy pills' so that you continue to take a pill every day. If you are someone who might forget, then this might be a good option for you. You can also run one pack of 21 straight into another so that you miss that withdrawal bleed if your bleed is due over a holiday or special event.

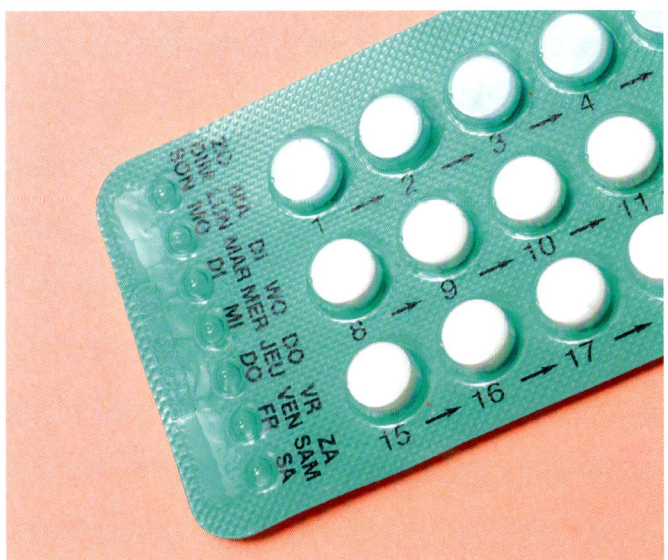

Lots of women worry that they may gain weight taking the combined pill, but research has shown this is not the case.

The pill can cause a rise in blood pressure. There is a very small increased risk of blood clots and this is mostly in women with a family history of blood clots, smokers, the very inactive or if you are very overweight.

You should not take the combined pill if you:

- Are significantly obese (body mass index greater than 35)
- Have high blood pressure
- Have a history of blood clots
- Have migraine with aura
- Have blood disorders that make you more prone to clotting
- Are breast feeding
- Have breast or liver cancer
- Have disease of the gallbladder
- Have a condition called SLE

The Mini Pill (progesterone only pill – POP)

This type of pill is taken every day without a break and works by thickening cervical mucus and thinning the lining of the womb. Most mini pills need to be taken within a three-hour window of the same time every day. Cerazette is a form of mini pill that also prevents ovulation and like the combined pill has a 12-hour window so may be more appropriate for you if your schedule is very changeable. Your bleeding may be less predictable on the mini pill and some women find their periods stop altogether.

The contraceptive patch

The contraceptive patch is basically the combined pill in patch form which is changed on the same day each week. The patch is about 5cm square. Some women find it can cause some skin irritation, but you can minimise this by rotating the site you use each week. The same rules as the COCP apply regarding who this form of contraception is not suitable for.

The contraceptive ring

This is a small clear ring about 5cm in diameter containing the same hormones as the COCP, so the same rules apply, but as this stays in place for three weeks at a time, women who find taking a pill every day a hassle, may prefer this option.

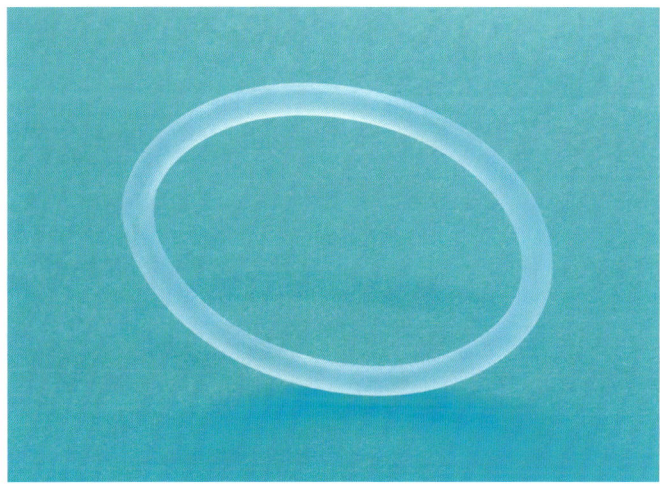

Long-acting reversible contraceptives

I think of these as the 'set and forget' contraceptives because once in place you don't need to think about contraception for weeks and in some cases years. They include:

Injections

Contraceptive injections contain progestogen are given every two or three months depending on the type. The most commonly used injection is given every 12 weeks and if you are more than a week late, you may be asked to do a pregnancy test to confirm that you are not pregnant before the next injection. This form of contraception can sometimes be associated with weight gain particularly in younger women (under 18) who are already overweight. Irregular bleeding can be an issue especially when the injection is first used.

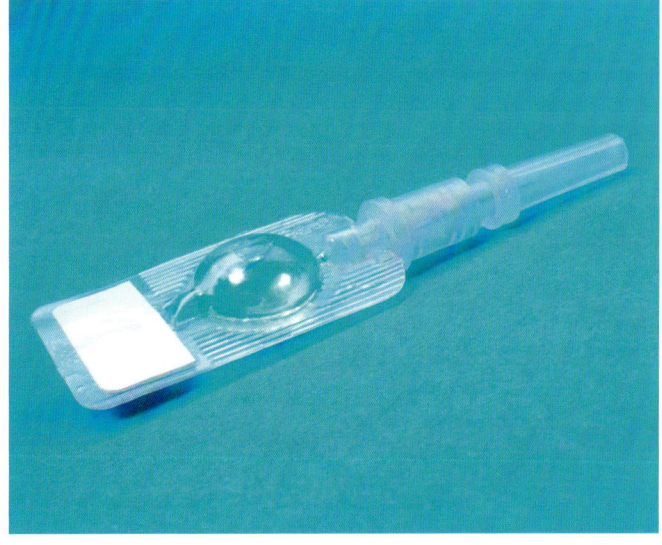

It is also possible to get side effects from the hormone, which include acne, hair loss, mood swings, loss of libido and headaches.

Long term it is possible that the injection can affect your oestrogen levels and put you at risk of osteoporosis (brittle bones). If you have other risk factors for this disease such as low weight, excess alcohol intake, a positive family history, long-term use of steroids, cigarette smoking or thyroid disease, then your doctor may suggest an alternative form of contraception.

There is no long-term risk to fertility but there can be a delay of up to a year when coming off the injection before periods start again and fertility is completely back to normal.

The contraceptive implant

This is small rod the size of a matchstick that is inserted under the skin of the arm under local anaesthetic. It slowly releases progestogen over a three-year period giving you effective contraception for all that time until it needs to be removed and replaced (again under local anaesthetic).

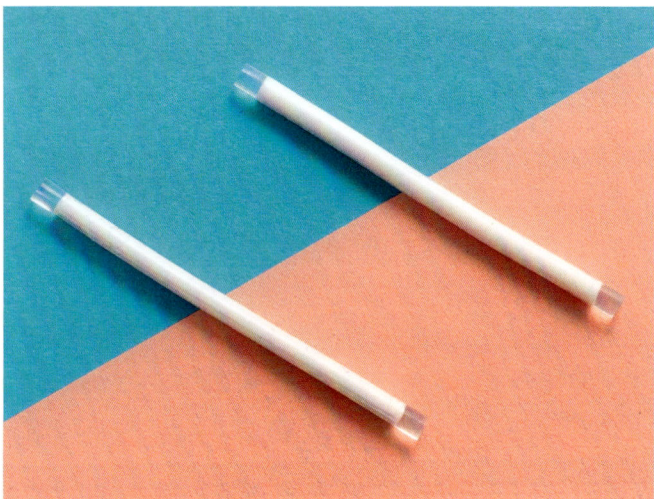

Intrauterine devices (Coils or IUDs)

I am a bit sad about the term 'coil', as I think it puts some women off. The truth is, when I show women coils, they are always surprised by how small they are. They are made of plastic or copper and can be fitted by Family Planning Clinics and some GP practices. There are lots of different types available, some of which will last for 10 years before needing to be replaced.

Some women find their periods are heavier with an IUD but some of this may also be because a lot of women go from using the COCP (where periods are lighter) to an IUD so we are not always comparing like with like.

They can also be used for emergency contraception (see below), in which case they can stay in place and be used as longer-term contraception.

The intrauterine system (IUS)

This is like a coil only it contains progestogen which is slowly released into the lining of the womb. It is fitted in the same way as a coil but it is slightly larger, so if you have never had children, they may use local anaesthetic to fit it. The total hormone absorbed into the body is similar to taking two mini pills in a week, so hormonal side effects are much less likely. It can cause erratic spotting for three to six months but after this a lot of women find their periods stop altogether. It needs replacing every three or five years depending on which brand you have fitted.

Natural contraception

Natural contraception requires you to be very in tune with your body and to be prepared to abstain from sex on your fertile days which can be as many as nine days a month.

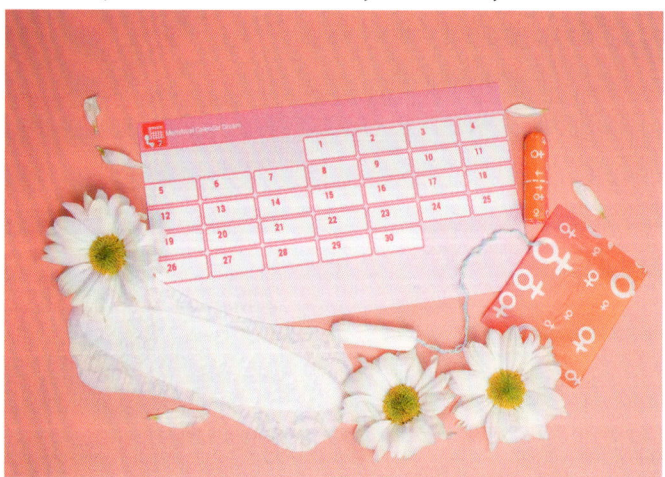

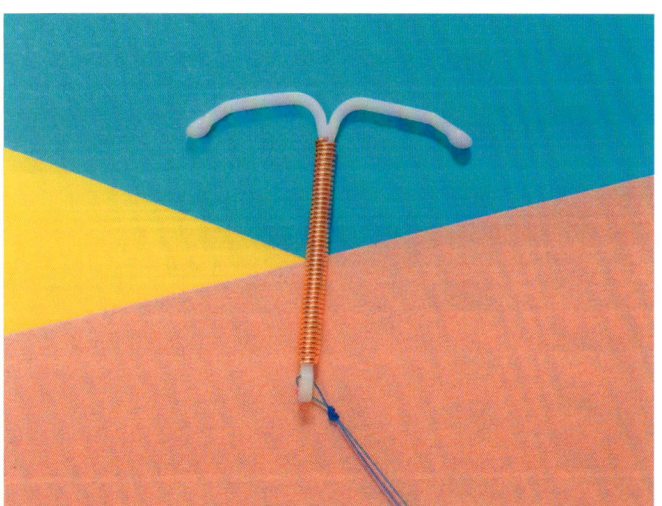

The signs you need to look for are:

- Body temperature – if you record your body temperature before you get out of bed each day and before you have anything to eat or drink, you will notice that at the time of ovulation your temperature will rise very slightly, about 0.2 degrees centigrade. This is when you are fertile. Your fertile time ends when your temperature has been higher for three days in a row.

- Cervical secretions – cervical secretions become clearer and wetter just before ovulation, a bit like the consistency of raw egg white. This is your fertile time. After ovulation the secretions become thicker and sticky. When they have been like this for three days you are no longer in your fertile phase.

- Cervical changes – Your cervix will feel slightly higher in the vagina and become softer and slightly open around the time of ovulation, which indicates your fertile time.

Emergency contraception

You can access free emergency contraception from Family Planning Clinics, GP surgeries, Sexual Health Clinics, Walk-in Centres, Minor Injuries Units, A&E and pharmacies although not all of these will offer the IUD option.

The emergency contraceptive pill ('morning-after' pill)

There are two types of emergency contraceptive pill. Levonelle can be used any time up to three days after unprotected sex and EllaOne can be used up to five days after unprotected sex.

The IUD

The IUD can be inserted up to five days after unprotected sex.

If you are still struggling to decide what contraception to use then speak to your GP. The Brook Contraception Tool can also help you work out the best method for you.

15 September 2022

The above information is reprinted with kind permission from Hidden Strength.
© 2024 Hidden Strength Holdings Ltd.

www.hiddenstrength.com

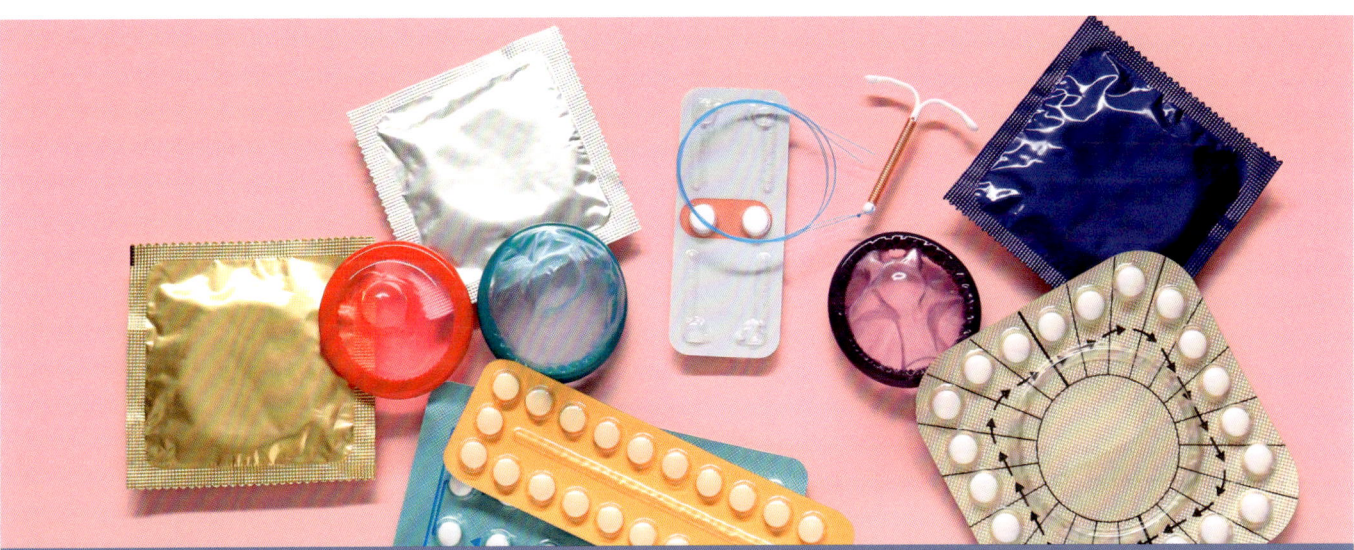

Where to get contraception

Contraception services are free and confidential on the NHS.

You can get contraception, including emergency contraception, for free from:

- Sexual health clinics, also called family planning or contraception clinics
- Some GP surgeries
- Some young people's services (call the national sexual health helpline on 0300 123 7123 for more information)

Getting the pill without a prescription

Some pharmacies offer the contraceptive pill for free without you needing to see a doctor or nurse for a prescription.

Where to buy contraception

You also do not need a prescription to buy:

- Condoms from pharmacies, supermarkets or online

- The emergency contraceptive pill (morning-after pill) from some pharmacies
- The progestogen-only pill (mini pill) from some pharmacies

Getting contraception if you're under 16

Contraception is free and confidential, including for young people under the age of 16.

The doctor or nurse will not tell anyone, including your parents or carer, unless they think you or someone else is at risk of harm.

12 February 2024

The above information is reprinted with kind permission from the NHS.
© Crown Copyright 2024
This information is licensed under the Open Government Licence v3.0
To view this licence, visit http://www.nationalarchives.gov.uk/doc/open-government-licence/

www.nhs.uk

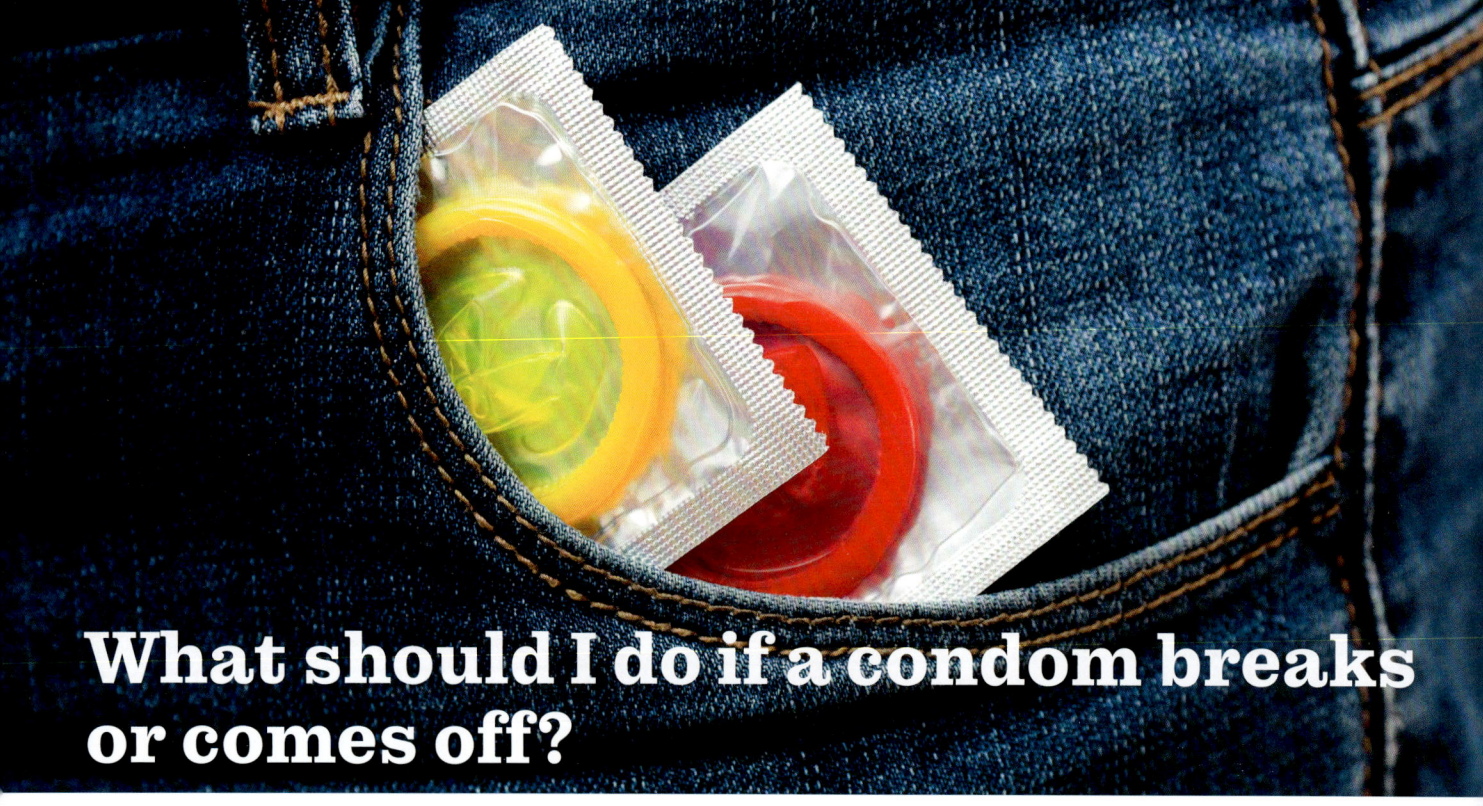

What should I do if a condom breaks or comes off?

Condoms, when used correctly, are very good at stopping STIs from getting passed on when having vaginal, anal or oral sex. They also do a brilliant job at preventing unwanted pregnancy. But it's an unfortunate fact that condoms can rip, break or come off completely, without you noticing. If this happens, here's what you should do to protect yourself and your partner.

Prevent pregnancy

If condoms are your only type of contraception, and you're not using another method like the pill, then emergency contraception can prevent pregnancy after sex. You need to get emergency contraception within 5 days (120 hours) of having sex for it to work effectively.

You can take emergency contraception pills (also known as morning-after pills) or have a non-hormonal coil fitted.

To get the morning-after pill, you can

- order online
- go to your local sexual health clinic, your GP, an NHS walk-in clinic or some pharmacies

Prevent STIs

Even a small tear in a condom can mean there's a chance of getting an STI. Infections do not always show symptoms, so the only way to be sure if you have one or not is with a test. But you should not test immediately – STIs take a few weeks to show up in tests, so if you do a test too soon, you will not get an accurate result.

If you were having sex with a new partner, you have not done a test for a while or you do not know the STI status of your partner, get tested at the right time to rule out common infections.

- Gonorrhoea and chlamydia tests are accurate 2 weeks (14 days) after sexual contact
- HIV tests is accurate at least 7 weeks (45 days) after sexual contact
- Syphilis test is accurate at 12 weeks (90 days) after sexual contact

Prevent HIV

If the condom breaking has put you at risk of HIV, for example you know your partner is HIV positive with a detectable viral load, you should look into getting PEP (post-exposure prophylaxis). This medicine can stop the virus from developing if you start it within 72 hours of sex.

You can get PEP from your local sexual health clinic or your nearest A&E department

Can you stop condoms from breaking?

Condoms are very rigorously tested to make sure they are strong, safe and keep you protected. Studies have found that only 0.4% of condoms break during sex. Using condoms correctly reduces the chances of tearing or breaking, this means:

- Do not use any lube or other products that have oil in. This can weaken condoms. So can the thrush treatment, clotrimazole cream
- Check the expiry date on the packaging and never use a condom that's past its expiry date.
- When you roll on a condom, pinch the tip to stop any air getting trapped
- Keep them away from heat and light, store them in a cool, dark place – like your bedside drawer
- Don't open them with anything sharp (like scissors, or your teeth)
- Get the right fit – condoms usually come in a range of sizes so check you are using the right size

7 February 2024

The above information is reprinted with kind permission from SH:24.

© 2024 SH:24

www.sh24.org.uk

Making informed decisions about taking the morning-after pill

In this guest blog, ellaOne®'s senior brand manager, Emma Marsh, highlights how education and access to emergency contraception can play a crucial role in helping prevent unplanned pregnancy.

Condom split? Missed pill? Caught in the moment? Whatever the reason, if you've had unprotected sex you could be at risk of pregnancy. But there is no need to panic and you certainly should not feel alone.

In research conducted by ellaOne®, 46% of women between the ages of 18–35 had unprotected sex in the last year, yet only 27% of those women took the morning-after pill. There are many reasons for three quarters (73%) of women skipping emergency contraception and risking unplanned pregnancy, including: embarrassment, misinformation and accessibility.

To reduce the risk of an unplanned pregnancy, it is wise to seek emergency contraception as soon as possible. You can either choose to take a morning-after pill, such as ellaOne®, or have a copper IUD fitted. The copper IUD, sometimes called the coil, is the most effective form of emergency contraception when inserted within five days of unprotected sex.

Any emergency contraceptive is more effective the sooner you use it, but when it comes to the morning-after pill, it's incredibly hard to separate the facts from the fiction.

In further research from ellaOne® that canvassed the views of over 1,000 British 18–35 year olds, the data revealed that 59% of people do not understand how emergency hormonal contraception (EHC) works by delaying ovulation (egg release), and over 40% thought the morning-after pill causes an abortion, which is incorrect. This highlights how and why so many young people struggle to get the right education and information when it comes to accessing emergency contraception when they need it most.

Where can you access the morning-after pill?

The morning-after pill can be accessed free of charge from a GP, or from your sexual health clinic. You can find your nearest sexual health clinic on the Brook website or you can also purchase the morning-after pill over the counter in pharmacies. ellaOne® is one type of morning-after pill available to buy from most pharmacies and can prevent pregnancy even right before ovulation (which is when risk of pregnancy is highest). ellaOne® can also be purchased online from ellaOne® Direct, for next-day home delivery.

ellaOne® contains ulipristal acetate and can be effective for up to five days (120 hours) after unprotected sex has taken place, but is most effective when taken as soon as possible. Other morning-after pills are effective within 72 hours after the event but are also most effective when taken as soon as possible. The morning-after pill is intended for use in the case of emergency and it is not meant to be a replacement for a regular method of contraception. If you often find yourself relying on emergency contraception, you may want to consider another contraceptive method. You can use this tool from Brook to help you understand what kinds of contraception may be best for you. Some daily contraceptives such as Hana®, a progestogen-only pill, are available to purchase in pharmacies or online without a prescription.

How does the morning-after pill work?

ellaOne® works by delaying ovulation so that any sperm in the reproductive system cannot find an egg to fertilise to help prevent pregnancy. When you have unprotected sex, sperm travel from the vagina, through the cervix and up the fallopian tubes where they wait for an egg. ellaOne® helps prevent or delay ovulation until all the sperm have died (five days), so there is no egg for them to fertilise and no pregnancy can take place.

If ovulation has already taken place, no morning-after pill will be effective

It is very hard to know when you are ovulating as your cycle can change from month to month and can be impacted by diet, stress and travel. By taking ellaOne® as soon as possible after unprotected sex, you reduce the risk of ovulating during that time.

The morning-after pill only works by preventing ovulation, it cannot cause an abortion and it will not have any effect in a case where an egg has already been fertilised.

13 September 2023

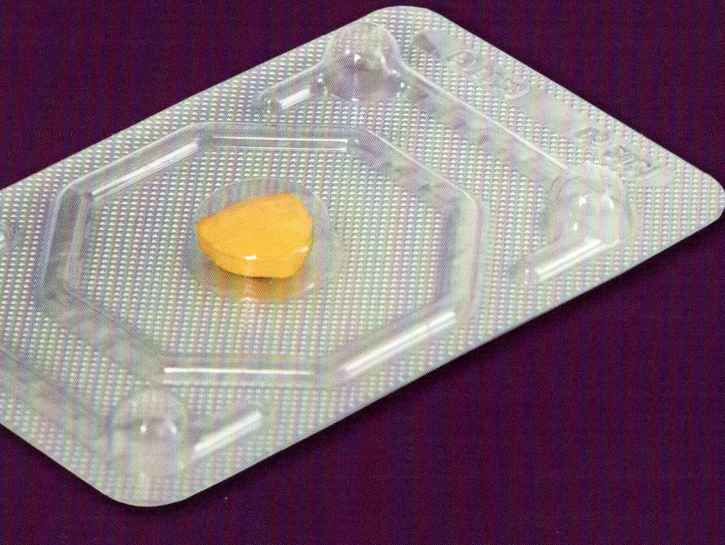

The above information is reprinted with kind permission from Brook Young People
© 2024 Brook Young People
www.brook.org.uk

Women in England to receive contraceptive pills at pharmacies

From next December 2023 women in England can get their contraceptive pills without contacting their GP first.

Thousands of women across England will soon be able to get the contraceptive pill at their local pharmacy without needing to contact their GP first.

From December 2023, pharmacies across the country will begin offering the new service for the first time, increasing choice for women in the ways in which they can access contraception.

The rollout is part of the Government and the NHS's primary care access recovery plan, which committed to making it quicker and easier for millions of people to access healthcare on their high street.

How does the service work?

Anyone needing the pill can access it through participating pharmacies without a referral from their GP, though they can be referred by their general practice or sexual health clinic.

The pharmacist will offer a confidential consultation and reach a shared decision with the person about their first supply of the pill, or the ongoing supply of their current oral contraception. The supply of oral contraception will be free.

What checks will I need?

For a combined oral hormonal contraception, a BMI and blood pressure measurement will need to be taken. These can be taken as part of the consultation within the pharmacy.

A person accessing the service may also offer their own weight, height and blood pressure measurements. Any self-reported measurements will need to be recorded as such.

Extensive training for pharmacists

Priya Littler is a pharmacist in Portsmouth and took part in a pilot of the service at the beginning of 2022. The pharmacy has seven branches across the city and all participated.

She said that the training for pharmacists was extensive, covering topics such as general consultation skills, the legal framework for prescribing combination and progesterone only contraception, as well as information around sexually transmitted infections and other areas that may come up during consultations.

Priya's pharmacy branch is on a high street near to a university campus, meaning she sees both students and young families.

'Some of our clients may find it difficult to get an appointment with their GP,' she said, 'so we wanted to make contraceptive pill services more accessible. It was also an interesting pilot for our teams to join, to expand their skills and knowledge.'

Consultations in minutes

Ben Morris, a pharmacist in Stoke-on-Trent, took part in a pilot of the scheme in October 2021, which gave local people the option to access their ongoing supply of oral contraception directly from their community pharmacist.

After undergoing the necessary clinical training, Ben began consultations in January 2022.

He says that when they first started, each would take around 10–15 minutes, but now they are comfortable with the system and what it involves, they are able to deliver the consultations in five or six minutes.

'Even with the combined pill, where we need to take blood pressure, height and weight, it's quick, including when people first register,' he said. 'When it's progesterone only, where we don't have to do the tests like with the combined pill, it's even quicker.

'It's basically a case of now we're used to it, we can deliver it more quickly. Where the patient consents, we also complete an anonymised returning patient message to the GP which adds about another five minutes.'

Easier access to contraception

Ben says anecdotal feedback was 'overwhelmingly positive'.

'The ease of access and our service delivery is also giving people more general confidence in us to use the other services we offer,' he said.

'Rather than having these patients arrange a GP appointment, surgeries are now simply passing queries directly to us.

'We're pleased that by working together, we have cemented their trust in us to deliver the confidential consultations in our private rooms and that we have the clinical expertise necessary to provide a repeat prescription.'

17 November 2023

The above information is reprinted with kind permission from the Prime Minister's Office.
© Crown Copyright 2024
This information is licensed under the Open Government Licence v3.0
To view this licence, visit http://www.nationalarchives.gov.uk/doc/open-government-licence/

www.gov.uk

Chapter 3

STIs

What is an STI?

Hey there! You might have heard about STIs in school, on TV, or maybe while eavesdropping on some hushed conversations. STI stands for Sexually Transmitted Infection, which can sound a bit scary, but knowledge is power, so let's dive in and demystify this topic together.

What exactly is an STI?

In simple terms, an STI is an infection you can get through sexual contact, which includes vaginal, anal, and oral sex. These infections are caused by viruses, bacteria, or parasites that are passed from one person to another during sexual activities. Sometimes, STIs are called STDs (Sexually Transmitted Diseases). The term 'disease' is used when an infection causes symptoms, although many people use STI and STD interchangeably.

How do you get STIs?

STIs are sneaky! You can't tell if someone has an STI just by looking at them. Often, people with STIs don't even know they're infected since they may not show any symptoms. So, having unprotected sex with someone who has an STI could mean you might get it too.

Remember, even if it's your first time, or if you've only had one partner, you can still get an STI. Some STIs, like herpes and HPV (human papillomavirus), can also be spread through skin-to-skin contact in the genital area. Also, a pregnant person can pass some STIs to their baby during childbirth or breastfeeding, but that's something you don't have to worry about just yet!

Common STIs among teenagers

There's a whole alphabet soup of STIs out there, but we'll highlight a few common ones:

- **HPV (human papillomavirus):** This is the most common STI and often has no symptoms. There are many different types of HPV; some can cause genital warts, while others can lead to cancers later in life.
- **Chlamydia:** This sneaky one often doesn't show symptoms either, but it can cause serious health issues if not treated.
- **Gonorrhoea:** Yep, another one with often no symptoms. It can infect the genitals, throat, and rectum.
- **Herpes:** This one shows up as blisters or sores on the genitals or mouth (cold sores). It's a lifelong infection, but symptoms come and go.
- **HIV (human immunodeficiency virus)**: Now this is serious. It attacks the immune system and can lead to AIDS (acquired immunodeficiency syndrome) if not treated.

Symptoms of STIs

Symptoms of STIs can vary wildly, but common signs might include:

- Sores, bumps, or blisters on the genitals or mouth
- Unusual discharge from the penis or vagina
- Itching or irritation around the genitals
- Pain during sex or while peeing
- Unusual bleeding, especially between periods

However, remember, many STIs don't show any symptoms at all!

Preventing STIs

The surefire way to prevent STIs is to abstain from sexual activity. But, let's be real; as teens start to explore their sexuality, it's essential to know how to protect yourself:

- Condoms: They're like super-heroes against STIs when used correctly every single time you have sex.
- Vaccination: Some STIs, like HPV, have vaccines that can prevent them – so getting vaccinated is a great step toward protection.
- Communication: Talk to your partner(s) about STIs and get tested regularly together. Being open about it is super important.
- Education: Learn about STIs. The more you know, the better equipped you'll be to protect yourself and your partners.

Getting tested for STIs

Testing for STIs isn't as scary as it sounds. It can be as easy as peeing in a cup or having a quick blood test. It's vital to get tested if you've had unprotected sex or if you're just starting a new relationship, even if you don't have any symptoms.

Sexual health clinics, and some GP's offer confidential testing and treatment. So, you can get checked without your parents or anyone else finding out.

Treatment for STIs

If you do happen to catch an STI, don't panic. Most STIs are treatable, and some are completely curable. Treatments can include antibiotics for bacterial STIs like chlamydia and gonorrhoea, and prescription creams or pills for viral STIs like herpes. HIV and some other STIs are not curable, but treatments can help manage symptoms and keep the virus under control.

10 signs you may have a sexually transmitted infection (STI)

Sexually transmitted infections (STIs) are a serious health issue, especially if left untreated. If you've had unprotected sexual intercourse or any intimate contact like touching or penetration, you may be at risk of contracting an STI. It's important to be aware of the warning signs, as early detection can help prevent complications. Here are 10 signs that you might have an STI:

1. Unusual discharge

If you notice a discharge that is different from your normal bodily fluids – whether it's from the vagina, penis, or anus – this could be a sign of an infection. The discharge might be thicker, have a strange colour, or smell different. If this happens, it's important to get it checked out as soon as possible.

2. Swelling, stinging, burning, or itching

Experiencing discomfort in your genital area, such as itching, burning, or swelling, is another common sign of an STI. This discomfort can occur around the penis, vagina, or anus. It might feel irritating when you sit, walk, or even wear tight clothes.

3. Lumps in the pubic or genital area

If you notice any lumps or bumps around your genital or anal area, they could be a sign of an STI. These lumps might appear in your pubic region, on your genitals, or around your anus. They can vary in size and might be painful or painless.

4. Painful urination or frequent urination

If it suddenly starts to hurt when you pee, or if you find yourself needing to pee more frequently than usual, you might have a urinary tract infection, which could be caused by an STI. Pain or a burning sensation when peeing is one of the most common signs of an infection.

5. Irregular or unusual bleeding

Unexpected bleeding from your genitals – whether it's from the vagina outside of your menstrual cycle or from the penis – should never be ignored. This could be a warning sign of an STI or another health issue that needs immediate attention.

6. Pelvic or testicular pain

Pain in the lower abdomen or around your testicles (for people with penises) or pelvis (for people with vaginas) can be a sign of an STI. This kind of discomfort could point to an infection that is affecting your reproductive organs, which may lead to serious complications if not treated.

7. Pain during sexual contact

If you feel pain during sex or any kind of sexual contact, it could mean there's an infection causing inflammation in your genital area. Pain during intercourse is often a sign that something isn't right and that your body is reacting to a problem like an STI.

8. Bumps, sores, or warts

Bumps, sores, or warts that appear around your penis, vagina, mouth, or anus are another key symptom of STIs, such as herpes or genital warts. These can vary in appearance, so it's important to see a healthcare provider if you notice anything unusual.

9. Flu-like symptoms

Feeling generally unwell – like having flu-like symptoms such as fever, chills, nausea, or fatigue – can sometimes be a sign of an STI. Your body may react to an infection by trying to fight it off, and this can make you feel sick overall.

10. No symptoms at all

It's crucial to remember that you might not experience any symptoms at all and still have an STI. Many infections, like chlamydia, can be asymptomatic, meaning you might feel completely fine but still be able to pass the infection to others. This is why regular testing is so important.

Why testing matters

STIs can take up to seven weeks to show up on a test after unprotected sex, even if you have no symptoms. If you think you may be at risk, speak to your GP or sexual health before getting tested, they will be able to advise when is the best time to get tested. However, if you do have symptoms, you should see a doctor immediately.

Remember, if you've had unprotected sex or notice any of these signs, the best thing you can do is get tested. Many STIs are treatable, but they can lead to serious health problems if ignored. Stay informed, stay safe, and protect yourself and your partners.

Activity

Create a poster with signs of how to spot a STI.

Include advice on what to do if you think you have a STI, such as information about your local sexual health or GUM clinic.

STIs: Get tested, get treated

In 2021 a total of 311,604 new STIs were diagnosed in England, an increase of 1,683 compared to 2020.

While still lower than pre-Covid-19 pandemic levels, the overall number of STIs newly diagnosed in England remains high, so it's important to get tested and prescribed effective treatment if needed. Ignoring STIs can lead to long-term problems, such as infertility.

Here we discuss and summarise the key findings from our report Sexually transmitted infections and screening for chlamydia in England, 2021 which we need to know to understand the risks, along with some simple steps we can take to stay in good sexual health.

Who is most at risk of STIs?

Everyone who has condomless sex with new or casual partners is at risk of catching an STI.

As in previous years, the highest rates of STI diagnoses were seen in gay, bisexual and other men who have sex with men (GBMSM); young people 15 to 24 years; and people of Black ethnicity.

Compared to people 25 and older, young people aged 15 to 24 years remain at the highest risk of the most common STIs, and this may be due to more frequent changes of sexual partners.

While the number (133,342) of new STI diagnoses in 2021 among young people aged 15 to 24 years decreased overall by 5.8% compared to 2020, reductions in testing during the Covid-19 pandemic may be behind this, prompting concerns that more infections could unknowingly be going untreated.

STI diagnoses in GBMSM increased between 2020 and 2021 – including diagnoses of gonorrhoea, chlamydia and syphilis.

Diagnoses of gonorrhoea increased by 9.0%, from 24,784 to 27,123, chlamydia increased by 5.5%, from 14,191 to 14,980, and diagnoses of infectious syphilis increased by 2.6%, from 5,118 to 5,254.

Compared to other ethnic groups, the rates of STI diagnoses remained highest among people of Black Caribbean ethnicity in 2021.

Previous research has found no unique clinical or behavioural factors explaining the higher rates of STI diagnoses among people of Black Caribbean ethnicity. This disparity is likely influenced by underlying social and economic factors and the role they play in the health inequalities experienced by this community.

HIV – what's the latest data telling us?

In 2021, new HIV diagnoses rose by 1%, to 2,955, with increases seen in GBMSM and heterosexual and bisexual women.

The proportion of those diagnosed late rose from 44% to 46%. The rise in late diagnoses is likely a consequence of the Covid-19 pandemic leading to reduced numbers of people testing in 2020, affecting heterosexual men and women in particular.

HIV testing is the route into accessing HIV pre-exposure prophylaxis (PrEP) which has been proven to reduce HIV transmission. If you are diagnosed with HIV, treatment is effective and people diagnosed promptly can expect long, healthy lives.

Effective treatment of HIV leads to undetectable levels of virus, which also means HIV cannot be passed on through sex ('undetectable = untransmittable' or 'U=U').

How can I protect myself against STIs?

STIs can pose serious consequences to your own health and that of your current or future sexual partners.

Using condoms is important to prevent spread of STIs and HIV, and is a key tool in looking after our sexual health and wellbeing.

If you are having sex with new or casual partners, use a condom and get tested – if you have any unusual symptoms, don't have sex until you are tested.

Get tested regularly for STIs

Regular testing for STIs and HIV is essential to maintain good sexual health.

Everyone should get an STI screen including an HIV test at least once a year if having condomless sex with new or casual partners – even if they don't have any symptoms.

Those at risk of STIs and HIV can access testing through sexual health services.

Many services offer online testing, which means people can order self-sampling kits using sexual health services' websites, take them in the privacy of their own home, send them off to a laboratory for testing and receive results either by text, phone call or post.

Local sexual health services can be found online at the NHS website.

If I test positive for an STI, where do I get treatment?

Sexual health services are free and confidential and offer treatment as well as testing for HIV and STIs.

Sexual health services also provide condoms, vaccination, HIV PrEP, and HIV post-exposure prophylaxis (PEP).

Information and advice about sexual health including how to access services is available at the NHS website and from the national sexual health helpline on 0300 123 7123.

4 October 2022

The above information is reprinted with kind permission from the UK Health Security Agency.

© Crown Copyright 2024

This information is licensed under the Open Government Licence v3.0
To view this licence, visit http://www.nationalarchives.gov.uk/doc/open-government-licence/

www.ukhsa.blog.gov.uk

Sexually transmitted infections found in 13-year-olds as cases hit record high

Cases of gonorrhoea, chlamydia and syphilis have all increased significantly, new figures show.

By Ella Pickover

Cases of gonorrhoea in England have reached record highs while children as young as 13 have been diagnosed with the sexually transmitted infection, new figures show.

The number of cases of chlamydia and syphilis have also dramatically increased, with the number of diagnosed cases of infectious syphilis at the highest level since just after the Second World War.

New UK Health Security Agency (UKHSA) figures show that overall there were 392,453 diagnoses of new STIs in England in 2022 – more than 1,000 every day and an increase of 23.8% compared with 2021.

While the rise in cases is, in part, linked to an increase in testing, health officials said the the sharp rise 'strongly suggests' there is more transmission of STIs in the population.

- Gonorrhoea diagnoses rose to to 82,592 in 2022, an increase of 50.3% compared with 2021 and the highest number of gonorrhoea diagnoses in any one year since records began in 1918.
- There were 50 cases of gonorrhoea diagnosed among 13– to 14-year olds.
- 537 over 65s were diagnosed with gonorrhoea in 2022 compared with 387 before the pandemic in 2019.
- Case rates in 2022 appeared to be highest in London for gonorrhoea. There were 383.4 cases of gonorrhoea diagnosed out of every 100,000 people in the capital compared with 68 per 100,000 in the Eastern England.
- Infectious syphilis diagnoses increased to 8,692 in 2022, the largest annual number since 1948.
- Chlamydia diagnoses increased by 24.3% from 160,279 diagnoses in 2021 to 199,233 in 2022.
- This includes 68,882 chlamydia diagnoses among people aged 15–24.

The UKHSA said people aged 15 to 24 are most likely to be diagnosed with STIs as it urged those who are having sex with new or causal partners to wear a condom and get tested regularly.

It said STIs are usually easily treated with antibiotics but many can cause serious health issues if left untreated.

Chlamydia and gonorrhoea can cause infertility and pelvic inflammatory disease, while syphilis can cause potentially

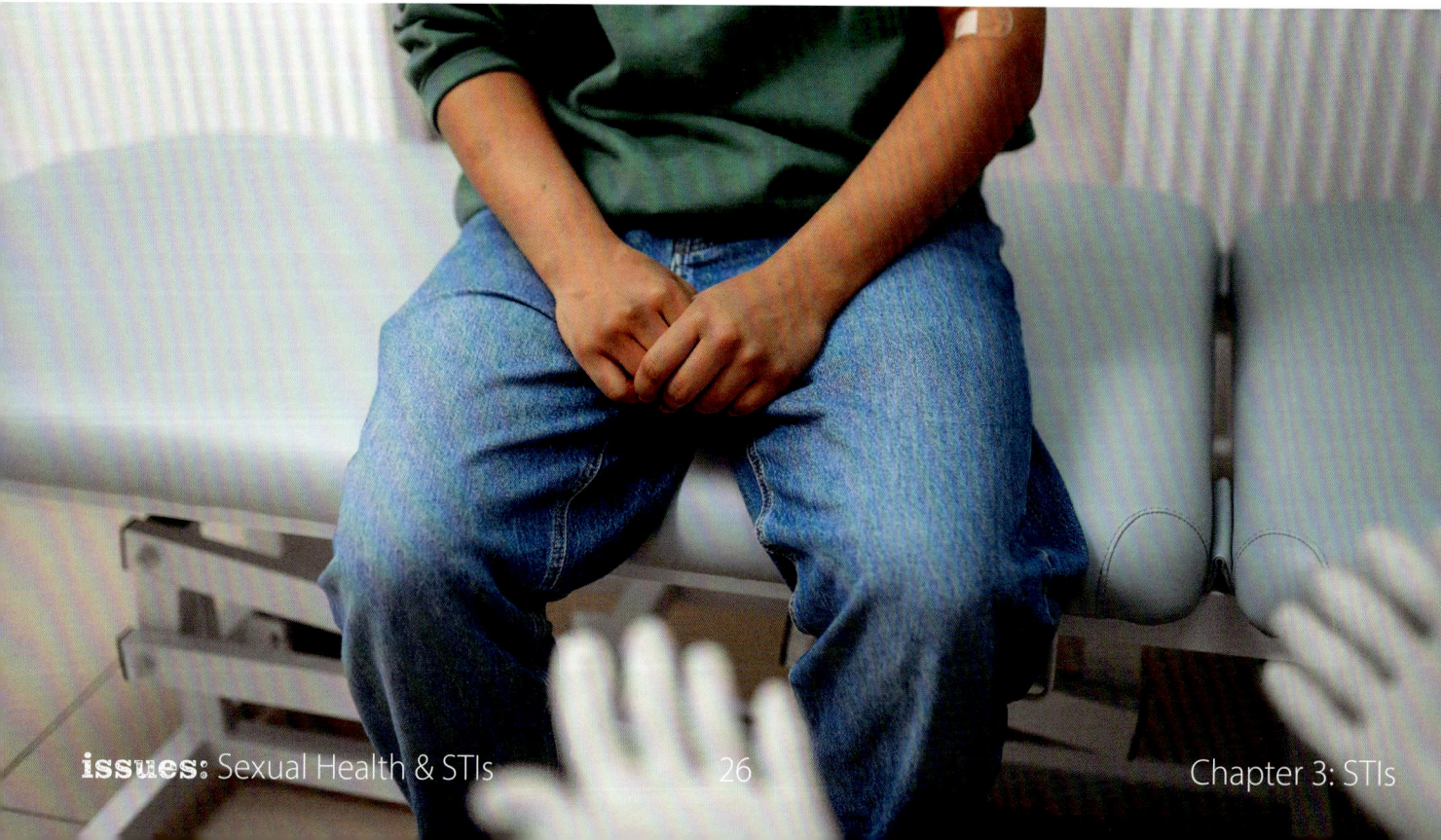

life-threatening problems with the brain, heart or nerves.

'We saw more gonorrhoea diagnoses in 2022 than ever before, with large rises, particularly in young people,' said Dr Hamish Mohammed, consultant epidemiologist at UKHSA.

'STIs aren't just an inconvenience – they can have a major impact on your health and that of any sexual partners.

'Condoms are the best defence but if you didn't use one the last time you had sex with a new or casual partner, get tested to detect any potential infections early and prevent passing them on to others.

'Testing is important because you may not have any symptoms of an STI.'

In 2022, there were 2,195,909 diagnostic tests for chlamydia, gonorrhoea, syphilis or HIV – 13.4% more than 2021.

Commenting on the figures, Richard Angell, chief executive of the sexual health charity Terrence Higgins Trust, said: 'The significant rise in sexually transmitted infections is a worrying testament to the fact that there is no vision or ambition for improving sexual health in England. We've seen cuts where we need to see investment, this has reduced our sexual health services to a minimal disease management process. This cannot continue.

'If this were any other set of health conditions, there would be outcry and we'd see rapid action and much-needed funding.

'Testing rates remain lower than pre-Covid-19, but the number of STIs being diagnosed are exceeding the high levels reported before the pandemic.

'In 2022, more than 1,000 STIs were diagnosed on average every day.

'Two years of social distancing resulted in a small drop in transmission rates but numbers are surging again because sexual health services and public health budgets have been cut to the bone.

'Until sexual health is properly resourced, we won't see the number of STIs heading in the right direction.'

He added: 'Year after year, the same groups are most impacted by STIs, including young people, gay and bisexual men, people living with HIV and those of Black Caribbean ethnicity. But nothing is being done to properly understand the impact of structural inequalities on poor sexual health, including racism, sexism, homophobia and transphobia.

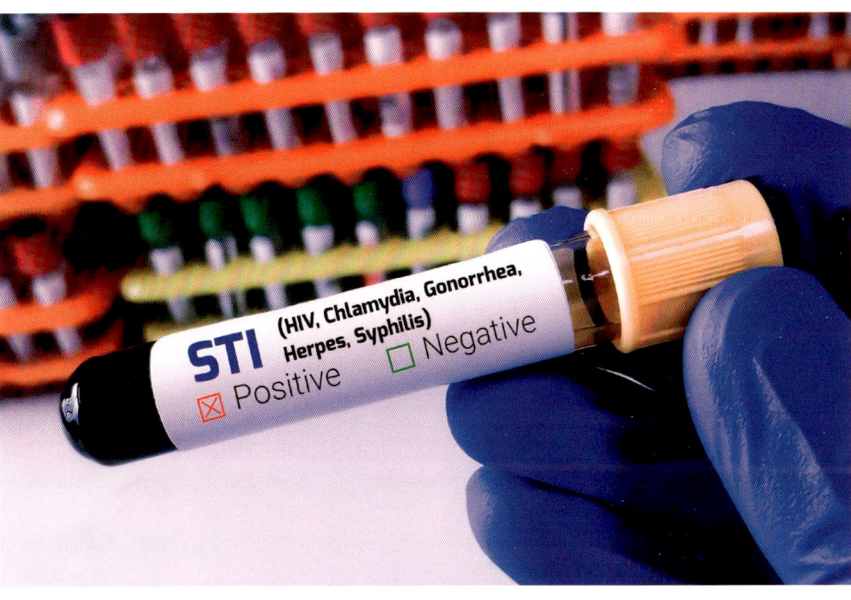

> **We've seen cuts where we need to see investment, this has reduced our sexual health services to a minimal disease management process**
>
> – Richard Angell, Terrence Higgins Trust

'The Government urgently needs to set out what good looks like for sexual health. We've been waiting four years for Government's sexual and reproductive health action plan and this latest data must come as a wake-up call to inspire action.'

David Fothergill, chairman of the Local Government Association's Community Wellbeing Board, said: 'Local council-commissioned sexual health services are at risk of breaking point, with rising demand coming at the same time as real-terms cuts to funding.

'It is encouraging to see more people visiting their local sexual health clinic, which is a testament to the work of councils with hard-to-reach communities in their areas, as well as the new cutting-edge treatments on offer.

'However, this is becoming increasingly unsustainable without a long-term increase in councils' public health grant, which goes towards funding vital sexual health services.

'The Government should ensure sexual and reproductive health funding is increased to levels which matches the increases local services have seen in demand. Investment in early intervention helps to save costs to the health service and prevents problems developing further down the line.'

6 June 2023

The above information is reprinted with kind permission from *The Independent*.
© independent.co.uk 2024

www.independent.co.uk

Guide to Sexually Transmitted Infections (STIs)

Chlamydia

Description: Chlamydia is a common sexually transmitted infection (STI) caused by the bacterium chlamydia trachomatis. It affects both men and women and can lead to serious health issues if left untreated, such as infertility in women. It is often referred to as a 'silent' infection because many people with chlamydia experience no symptoms, allowing it to spread unknowingly.

Signs or symptoms: Symptoms, when they do appear, may include abnormal discharge from the vagina or penis, pain during urination, or discomfort during sex. Women may also experience abdominal pain or bleeding between periods.

Diagnosis: Chlamydia is diagnosed through a urine test or a swab from the affected area (e.g., cervix, urethra).

Treatments: Chlamydia is easily treated with antibiotics, usually azithromycin or doxycycline.

Genital warts

Description: Genital warts are caused by certain strains of the human papillomavirus (HPV). They appear as small bumps on the genital or anal area and can vary in size and shape. Though not typically dangerous, they can cause discomfort and may recur after treatment.

Signs or symptoms: Visible warts around the genital or anal region, itching, or discomfort during sex. In some cases, warts may be so small they are not easily noticed.

Diagnosis: A doctor can diagnose genital warts by visually examining the affected area. In some cases, a biopsy may be needed for confirmation.

Treatments: Treatment may involve topical creams, freezing (cryotherapy), or minor surgery to remove the warts. However, the virus may remain in the body even after treatment.

Prevention: Vaccination against HPV, practising safe sex, and regular health check-ups can reduce the risk of genital warts. Using condoms can also help but may not fully protect against warts since they may occur in areas not covered by the condom.

Gonorrhoea

Description: Gonorrhoea is an STI caused by the bacterium neisseria gonorrhoeae. It primarily affects the genital tract, but it can also infect the rectum and throat. Untreated gonorrhoea can lead to serious health complications, including infertility and increased risk of HIV.

Signs or symptoms: Symptoms may include a burning sensation when urinating, unusual discharge from the penis or vagina, or pain and swelling in one or both testicles in men. Women may also experience pelvic pain and bleeding between periods.

Diagnosis: Gonorrhoea is diagnosed through a urine test or a swab from the affected area, such as the cervix, urethra, throat, or rectum.

Treatments: Gonorrhoea is treated with antibiotics, typically a combination of an injection and oral antibiotics.

Herpes

Description: Herpes is a viral infection caused by the herpes simplex virus (HSV). There are two types: HSV-1, which usually causes oral herpes (cold sores), and HSV-2, which causes genital herpes. Once contracted, the virus remains in the body, and outbreaks can occur over time.

Signs or symptoms: Symptoms include painful blisters or sores around the mouth or genital area, itching, and discomfort. Some people may experience flu-like symptoms during an initial outbreak.

Diagnosis: Herpes can be diagnosed through a physical examination, a swab of the sores, or a blood test that detects the virus.

Treatments: There is no cure for herpes, but antiviral medications can reduce the severity and frequency of outbreaks.

Prevention: Using condoms and avoiding sexual contact during an active outbreak can help prevent the spread of herpes.

HIV & AIDS

Description: HIV (human immunodeficiency virus) attacks the immune system, weakening the body's ability to fight infections and diseases. If untreated, it can lead to AIDS (acquired immunodeficiency syndrome), the most severe phase of the virus. HIV is transmitted through contact with infected blood, semen, vaginal fluids, or breast milk.

Signs or symptoms: Early symptoms of HIV resemble flu-like symptoms, such as fever, fatigue, and sore throat. Over time, without treatment, HIV can progress to AIDS, leading to weight loss, recurring infections, and serious health complications.

Diagnosis: HIV is diagnosed through blood tests that detect the virus or the antibodies the body produces in response to it.

Treatments: Although there is no cure for HIV, antiretroviral therapy (ART) can effectively manage the virus, allowing people to live long, healthy lives.

Prevention: HIV can be prevented by using condoms, getting tested regularly, and avoiding sharing needles. Pre-exposure prophylaxis (PrEP), a daily medication, can also help prevent infection in high-risk individuals.

Human papillomavirus (HPV)

Description: HPV is a group of viruses that affect the skin and mucous membranes. It is the most common STI and is transmitted through skin-to-skin contact during sexual activity. While many HPV infections clear up on their own, some strains can lead to genital warts or cancer, particularly cervical cancer.

Signs or symptoms: Most people with HPV do not show any symptoms. Some may develop genital warts, while others may not notice any signs until they develop complications like cancer.

Diagnosis: HPV is often detected through cervical screening (Pap smears) in women. There is no specific test for HPV in men, but doctors can diagnose genital warts visually.

Treatments: There is no cure for HPV, but the immune system often clears the infection on its own. Treatments are available for the symptoms, such as removal of genital warts.

Prevention: HPV vaccines are highly effective in preventing infection with cancer-causing strains. Safe sex practices, including condom use, also lower the risk of HPV transmission.

Mycoplasma genitalium

Description: Mycoplasma genitalium is a bacterial STI that can infect the urethra, cervix, and reproductive organs. It is often overlooked due to its similarity to other STIs, but untreated infections can lead to serious reproductive health problems.

Signs or symptoms: Symptoms may include painful urination, abnormal genital discharge, and pelvic pain in women. Many people experience no symptoms, which makes it easy to spread.

Diagnosis: Mycoplasma genitalium is diagnosed through a specific nucleic acid amplification test (NAAT), as it is not detected by standard STI screenings.

Treatments: The infection is treated with antibiotics, but some strains of the bacteria have developed resistance, making treatment more complex.

Pubic lice

Description: Pubic lice, also known as 'crabs,' are tiny parasitic insects that infest the hair in the pubic region. They are spread through close personal contact or sharing clothing and bedding with an infested person.

Signs or symptoms: Intense itching in the pubic area, visible lice or eggs on the hair, and small blue spots or sores caused by bites are common symptoms.

Diagnosis: A visual inspection of the pubic hair can usually confirm the presence of pubic lice.

Treatments: Over-the-counter lotions and shampoos containing permethrin or pyrethrin can treat pubic lice. Washing clothing and bedding in hot water is also essential to prevent reinfestation.

Scabies

Description: Scabies is a skin condition caused by tiny mites that burrow into the skin to lay eggs. It is highly contagious and can be spread through prolonged skin-to-skin contact or sharing clothing or bedding.

Signs or symptoms: Intense itching, especially at night, and a rash with small, raised red bumps are typical symptoms. The mites often burrow in folds of skin, such as between fingers, around the waist, or in the genital area.

Diagnosis: Scabies is diagnosed through a physical examination and sometimes a skin scraping to look for mites under a microscope.

Treatments: Topical creams or lotions, such as permethrin, are applied to the skin to kill the mites. All close contacts and household members should also be treated, even if they don't show symptoms.

Syphilis

Description: Syphilis is a bacterial STI caused by treponema pallidum. It progresses through stages, beginning with sores and potentially leading to severe complications like brain, nerve, or heart damage if left untreated.

Signs or symptoms: In the early stage, syphilis causes painless sores at the site of infection. If untreated, it can progress to a rash, fever, and swollen lymph nodes. In later stages, it can cause serious health problems.

Diagnosis: A blood test can diagnose syphilis by detecting antibodies to the bacteria. In some cases, a sample from a sore can be tested.

Treatments: Syphilis is treated with antibiotics, usually penicillin. Early treatment is crucial to prevent complications.

Trichomonas

Description: Trichomonas, also known as trichomoniasis, is a common STI caused by a parasite called trichomonas vaginalis. It primarily affects the genital area, but many people with trichomonas show no symptoms.

Signs or symptoms: When symptoms do occur, they may include itching or burning in the genital area, pain during urination, or unusual discharge from the penis or vagina.

Diagnosis: Trichomonas is diagnosed through a lab test of a swab or urine sample that detects the parasite.

Treatments: Trichomonas is easily treated with antibiotics, usually a single dose of metronidazole or tinidazole.

Yeast infection

Description: A yeast infection, also known as candidiasis, is caused by an overgrowth of a fungus called candida in the genital area. Although not an STI, yeast infections can develop after sexual contact due to changes in the vaginal environment.

Signs or symptoms: Symptoms include itching, burning, and thick, white vaginal discharge. Some women may also experience pain during urination or sex.

Diagnosis: Yeast infections can be diagnosed through a physical examination and a swab of the affected area, which is tested for fungal growth.

Treatments: Antifungal medications, available over-the-counter or by prescription, are used to treat yeast infections. These can be taken orally or applied directly to the affected area.

Prevention: Wearing breathable underwear, avoiding overly tight clothing, and maintaining proper hygiene can help prevent yeast infections. Reducing sugar intake and avoiding unnecessary use of antibiotics may also be beneficial.

STI myths

In today's world, being informed about sexually transmitted infections (STIs) is crucial for everyone, especially teenagers. There's a lot of misinformation out there, so let's debunk some common myths and arm you with the truth.

Can STIs be transmitted through condoms?

Condoms are your best defence against STIs when used correctly every single time you have sex. However, no method is 100% infallible. STIs like herpes or HPV, which spread through skin-to-skin contact, can still be transmitted through areas not covered by the condom. So, while condoms significantly reduce the risk, they can't eliminate it completely.

Can you transmit an STI through kissing?

While most STIs do not easily spread through kissing, there are exceptions, such as herpes simplex virus (cold sores) and cytomegalovirus. These can indeed be transmitted through simple acts like kissing. However, more severe STIs, like HIV, require more intimate body fluid exchanges than kissing usually involves.

Can STIs be caught from toilet seats?

This is a prevalent myth. The reality is that STIs are primarily transmitted through sexual activity. The bacteria and viruses that cause these infections cannot survive for long on the surface of a toilet seat, so it's incredibly unlikely to contract an STI this way.

Can STIs be transmitted through sharing towels?

Similar to the toilet seat myth, the chance of contracting an STI through sharing towels is exceedingly low. Most STI-causing bacteria and viruses do not live long outside the human body, making transmission via a towel very unlikely.

However, it is possible to spread scabies and pubic lice through shared towels, bedding or clothing.

Can you transmit STIs without ejaculating?

Yes, you can. Many STIs, including chlamydia and gonorrhoea, can be transmitted through pre-ejaculate fluid. Additionally, skin-to-skin contact diseases like HPV and herpes can be spread without ejaculation. It's essential to protect yourself and your partner every time.

Can STIs be transmitted through breastfeeding?

Certain STIs, like HIV, can indeed be transmitted from mother to child through breastfeeding. However, most other STIs cannot be spread this way. Mothers who are living with STIs should consult with their healthcare providers to find safe ways to feed their babies.

Can STIs be transmitted through oral sex?

Yes, STIs can be transmitted through oral sex. Many people wrongly assume that oral sex is risk-free, but infections like gonorrhoea, syphilis, and herpes can be passed through the mouth, throat, and genitals during oral activities. Using barriers like condoms or dental dams during oral sex can help reduce this risk.

Will an STI go away by itself?

Depending on the STI, the outcome can vary. Bacterial STIs like chlamydia and syphilis require antibiotic treatment and will not go away on their own. Viral STIs, such as herpes and HIV, have no cure, but their symptoms can be managed with medication. It's essential to get tested and seek treatment if you believe you may have an STI.

Does the 'pull out' method prevent STIs and pregnancy?

The 'pull-out' method, where the male partner withdraws before ejaculation, is not an effective way to prevent STIs or pregnancy. Pre-ejaculate fluid can contain STI pathogens and sperm, so transmission and conception can still occur even without full ejaculation. For STI and pregnancy prevention, more reliable methods like condoms should be used.

Being informed and practicing safe sex are the best ways to protect yourself and your partners from STIs. If you have any concerns or show symptoms of an STI, don't hesitate to consult a healthcare provider. Your health and wellbeing are too important to rely on myths and misinformation.

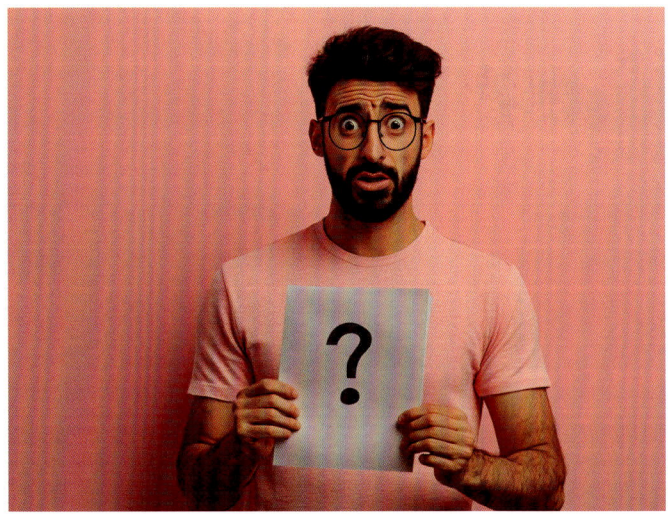

Anonymous Questions

Your teacher will have a box for anonymous questions, write your question on a piece of paper and place it in the box.

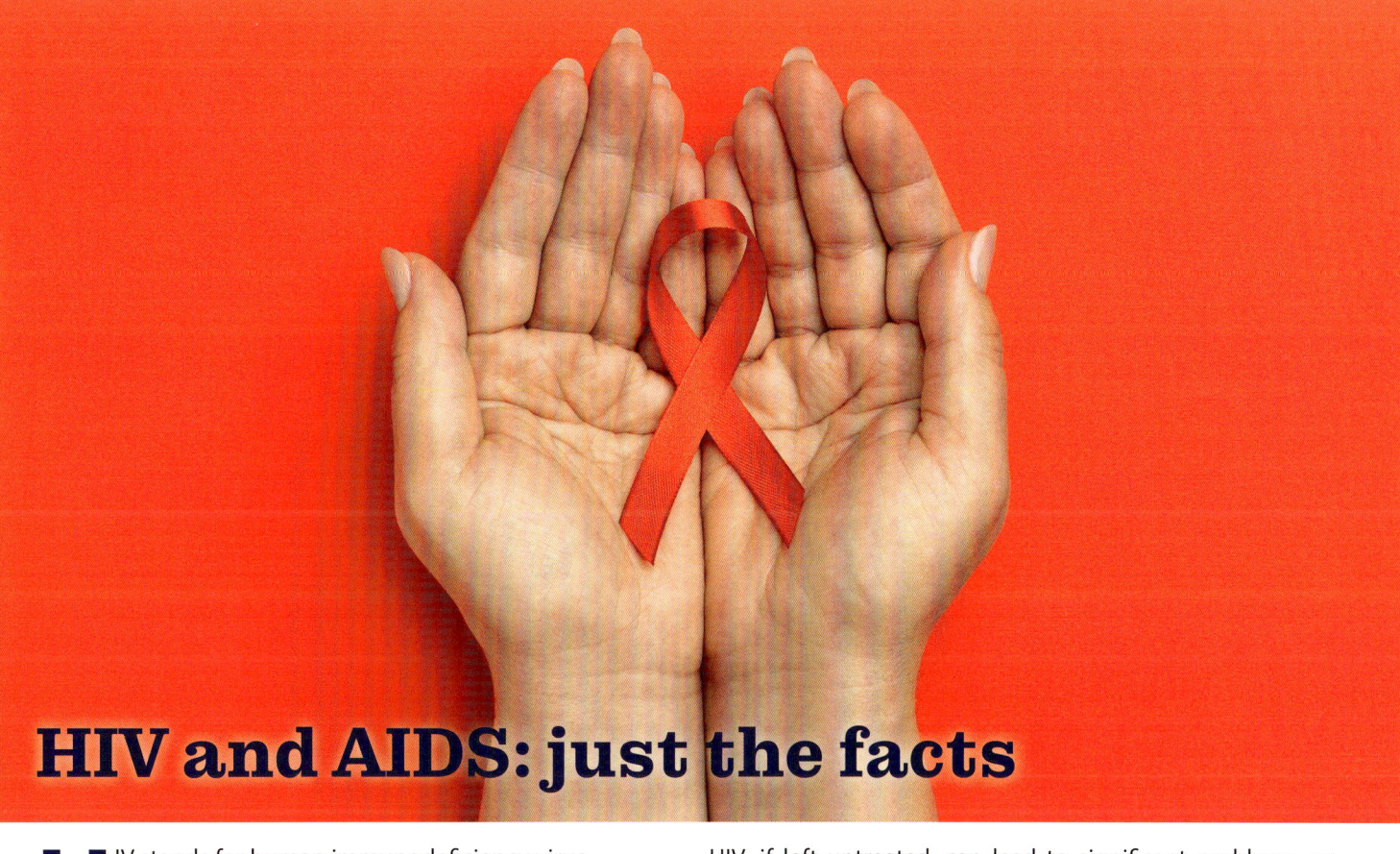

HIV and AIDS: just the facts

HIV stands for human immunodeficiency virus. It is a virus that damages cells in the immune system that work to fight infections.

AIDS stands for acquired immune deficiency syndrome. You suffer this as a result of long-term damage to the immune system caused by HIV when left untreated.

How can you get it?

HIV can be transmitted from one person to another via unprotected vaginal or anal sex.

When someone has HIV, the virus is present within their bodily fluids including semen, blood and anal fluids. It CANNOT be spread through contact with urine, saliva or sweat.

HIV can also be transmitted through the sharing of items that have touched blood, including needles.

In females infected with HIV, the virus can be transmitted from mother to baby during pregnancy.

Symptoms

HIV does not often have significant symptoms – this can make it difficult to know if you have been infected.

Testing

It is very important if you have had unprotected sexual intercourse and you think you may have HIV, or any other sexually transmitted disease, to get tested as soon as possible. To be tested for HIV (or any other sexually transmitted disease), visit:

- Your GP surgery
- A sexual health or GUM clinic.

This is important so you can begin treatment early if you test positive, which can reduce the risk of you becoming more unwell and transmitting the virus to others.

HIV, if left untreated, can lead to significant problems, so early treatment can prevent HIV developing into an AIDS-type illness.

Treatment

At present there is no cure for HIV, but there are medicines that enable people with the virus to live a near to normal life.

Tablets are used to treat HIV and work by stopping the virus multiplying in the body. This protects the immune system from being damaged.

Many people with diagnosed HIV will be treated with a combination of different medicines, these will be prescribed by a doctor and will help to build the body's resistance to HIV.

Effective HIV treatment can reduce the level of the virus in the body below the test levels, making HIV undetectable. This reduces the risk of transmitting HIV to others.

Remember...

You can prevent or reduce the risk of catching HIV by:

- Using a condom for sexual intercourse
- Being prescribed medication to protect those without HIV from infection. This medication does not protect against other sexually transmitted infections.

14 April 2021

The above information is reprinted with kind permission from the Health for Teens/NHS.

© Crown Copyright 2024

This information is licensed under the Open Government Licence v3.0
To view this licence, visit http://www.nationalarchives.gov.uk/doc/open-government-licence/

OGL

www.healthforteens.co.uk

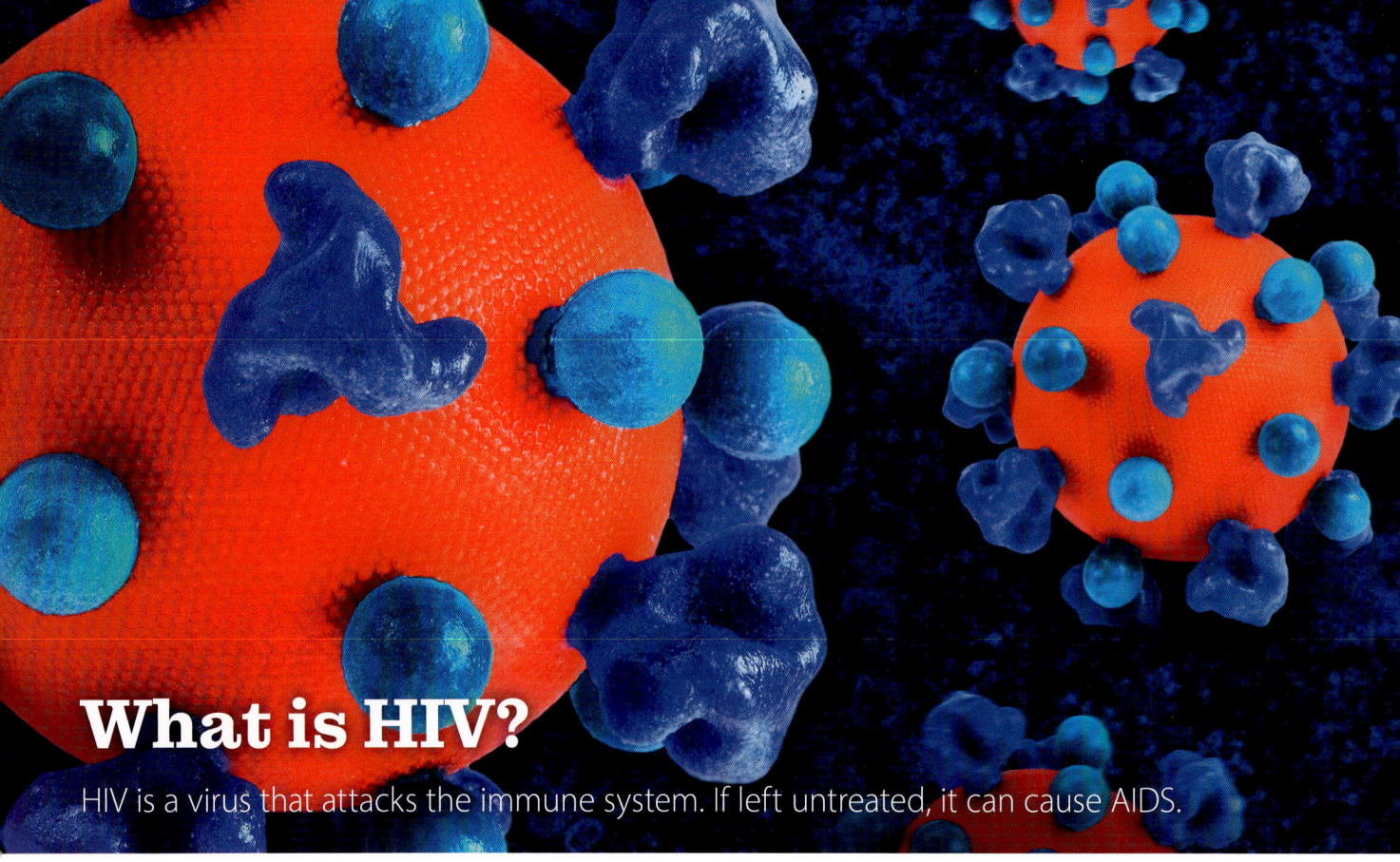

What is HIV?

HIV is a virus that attacks the immune system. If left untreated, it can cause AIDS.

Human immunodeficiency virus (HIV) is a virus that infects humans and attacks the immune system.

The final stage of HIV infection is acquired immunodeficiency syndrome (AIDS), which can be life-threatening.

There is currently no cure for HIV, but infections can be managed through regular clinical monitoring and antiretroviral treatments.

What is HIV?

HIV, or human immunodeficiency virus, is a virus that damages the cells of the immune system, weakening its ability to fight everyday infections.

Specifically, HIV attacks the CD4 T-cells, which are key immune cells involved in fighting infection and disease.

Destroying these immune cells leaves individuals open to various infections and the development of certain cancers.

What is AIDS?

Acquired immunodeficiency syndrome (AIDS) is the final stage of HIV infection. This is when the immune system has been diminished to the point that the body can no longer fight life-threatening infections.

People who have HIV are diagnosed with AIDS when their CD4 T-cell count is very low:

- a normal CD4 count ranges from 500–1,000 CD4 T-cells/mm3
- a CD4 count of fewer than 200 CD4 T-cells/mm3 qualifies for a diagnosis of AIDS.

With early detection of HIV and modern treatments for the infection, HIV infections can be managed to avoid them progressing to AIDS.

For example, antiretroviral therapy (or ART) suppresses the replication of the virus inside the body. This allows the immune system to repair itself and prevent further damage.

How is HIV transmitted?

HIV is found in some bodily fluids and can be transmitted:

- through unprotected sex
- by sharing of needles used to inject drugs
- from an HIV-positive mother to her child during childbirth or breast feeding.

HIV cannot be spread through sweat, urine or touching an infected person.

If a person with HIV is taking antiretroviral treatment, their virus levels ('viral load') can be reduced to be so low that the virus cannot be passed on. This is sometimes called 'U=U', for 'undetectable = untransmissible'.

Most people taking HIV treatment reach 'U=U' within six months of starting the treatment.

What are the symptoms of HIV?

Symptoms of HIV vary depending on the individual and the stage of HIV infection.

Early stage

2–4 weeks after infection, people with HIV tend to display flu-like symptoms, such as fever, swollen glands and sore throat.

This is the body's natural response to the HIV infection as it tries to fight it off.

Generally, this stage lasts from a few days to several weeks.

Latent stage

The disease moves into a 'latency' period where the virus continues to grow in the individual but without causing any symptoms.

If the infection is left untreated, the latent period lasts an average of 10 years in people with HIV.

For individuals given antiretroviral therapy (ART), the latent stage may last for several decades because this treatment helps to keep the virus under control, preventing it from progressing to the next stage, AIDS.

Progression to AIDS

If an individual is not taking any medication for their HIV, the virus will eventually weaken the body's immune system to the point that symptoms arise again.

Symptoms are much more profound than in the early stage and include rapid weight loss, extreme tiredness and memory loss.

This stage of HIV infection also leaves the body vulnerable to 'opportunistic' infections, which take advantage of the body's weakened immune state.

Opportunistic infections can be localised (meaning they only affect one part of the body) or systemic (meaning they have spread to other parts of the body).

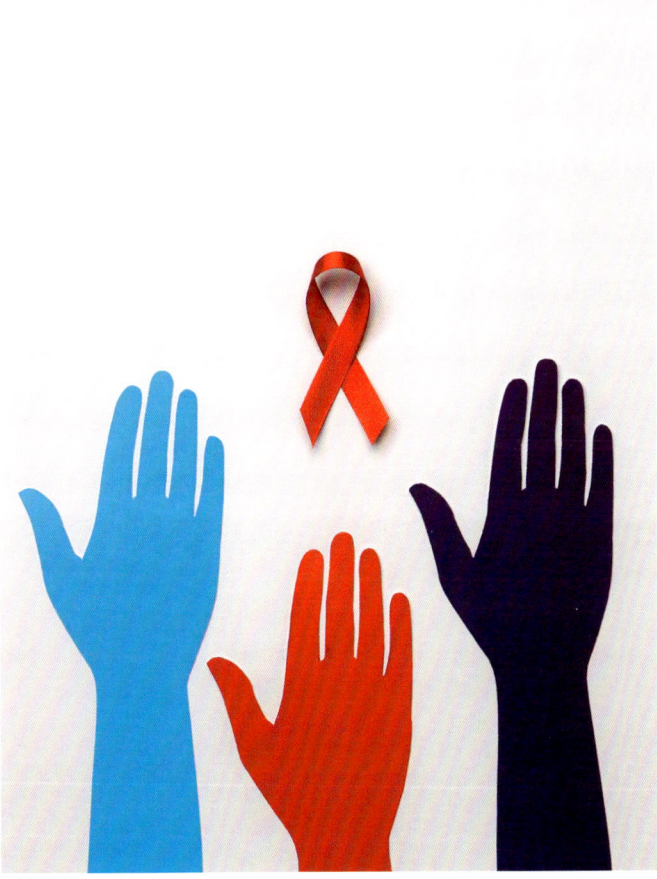

Examples of opportunistic infections include:

- Tuberculosis (TB): for people living with HIV, tuberculosis infections are very serious and are the leading cause of death. This is because people with HIV have a weakened immune system, so tuberculosis infections can quickly develop into disease if left untreated.

- Kaposi's sarcoma: is a rare form of cancer caused by human herpesvirus 8. Sarcomas develop primarily in the muscle, bone, nerves, tendons, blood vessels and fatty and fibrous tissue. Kaposi's sarcoma appears as red or purple lesions on the body and in the mouth but can also damage internal organs. Treatment includes surgery to remove small skin lesions or chemotherapy and radiotherapy if the disease has progressed.

- Toxoplasmosis: is caused by the parasite toxoplasma gondii, which is carried by cats and birds. It can cause mild flu-like symptoms but can also cause serious problems in the brain and eyes in HIV patients with low CD4 T-cell counts.

- Cytomegalovirus (CMV): is a human herpesvirus that is transmitted in bodily fluids and in most cases causes no symptoms or flu-like symptoms. Once infected, the virus never leaves the body but can re-emerge if the immune system is weakened. It can affect the eyes, lungs and digestive system causing inflammation.

If a person with HIV develops one or more of these opportunistic infections, it may indicate that their HIV infection has progressed to AIDS.

How is HIV managed?

If a person has been exposed to HIV, it's possible to take post-exposure prophylaxis (PEP) to stop the infection. This must be taken within 72 hours of exposure to be effective.

There is currently no cure for HIV, but infections can be managed through regular clinical monitoring and antiretroviral treatments.

These treatments control the HIV infection and prevent it progressing to AIDS.

HIV-infected people who manage their infections with antiretroviral treatments are able to live long and healthy lives.

The above information is reprinted with kind permission from Your Genome, part of Wellcome Connecting Science.

© 2024 Your Genome

www.yourgenome.org

Myths about HIV

Common misconceptions about HIV that can stop people from getting tested, from accessing treatment and from living well with HIV.

Since the 1980s, so much has changed about HIV, but myths and stigma still exist. Some of the myths are about how HIV is passed on, where HIV came from, and HIV treatment and the reality of living with HIV today.

These myths can stop people from getting tested, from accessing treatment and from living well with HIV. Stigma can cause discrimination and unfair treatment of people living with HIV.

What are common misconceptions about HIV?

1. 'HIV and AIDS are the same thing'

HIV is the name of a virus. AIDS (what we now call late stage or advanced HIV) is the name for a collection of illnesses caused by this virus.

You can't get an AIDS diagnosis unless you're already HIV positive, but many people who have HIV will never have AIDS. This is because advances in HIV treatment mean that HIV is now a long-term manageable condition.

2. 'HIV is a death sentence'

Before advances in HIV treatment, someone diagnosed with HIV in the 1980s and early 1990s may have only been given a few years to live. But today people living with HIV can live long healthy lives, if they are on treatment.

People with HIV can expect to live as long as their HIV negative peers. We are now seeing the first generation of HIV positive people growing old, living with HIV. In fact, the over 50s are the fastest growing group of people living with HIV. The challenge is now to support people to live well with HIV as they get older.

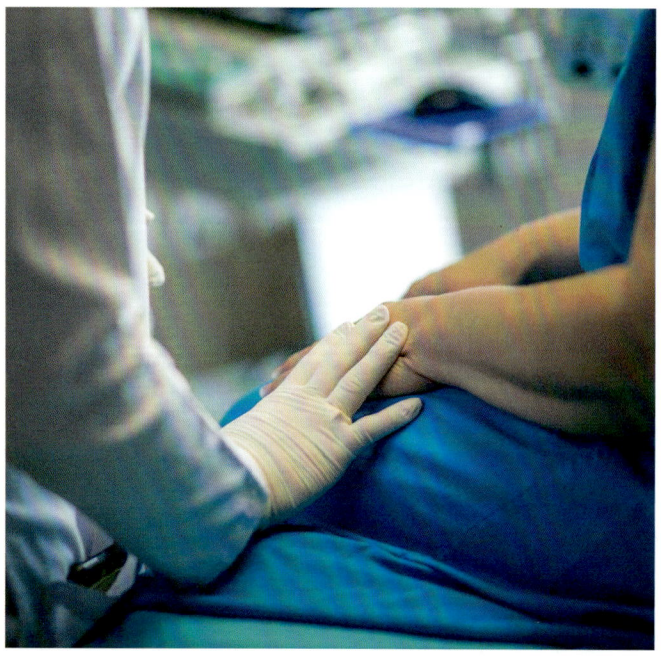

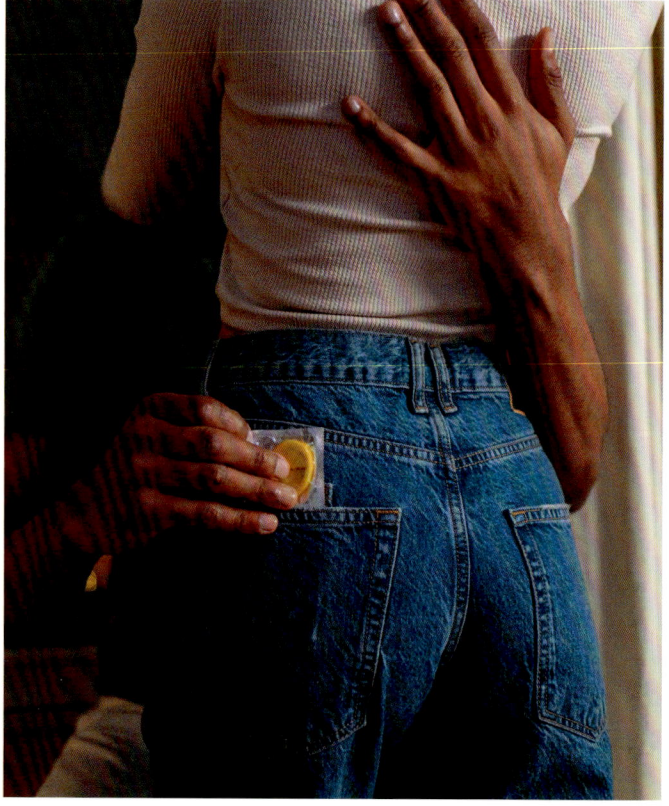

3. 'If you have sex with someone living with HIV, you will get HIV too'

People taking effective HIV treatment cannot pass on HIV through sex.

Effective treatment reduces the amount of the virus (your viral load) to very low, undetectable levels. Being undetectable means the level of HIV in your blood is so low, it can't be detected by the tests used to measure viral load and this means you cannot pass on the virus.

4. 'People with HIV can pass it on to others during everyday social contact'

HIV can only be passed on when one person's body fluids (e.g., blood, semen and fluids from the vagina, but not saliva) get inside another person's body. HIV is transmitted by vaginal/frontal sex, anal sex, oral sex (though very rarely), and sharing injecting equipment. A person living with HIV can't pass on the virus if their viral load is undetectable.

The virus cannot be transmitted by kissing, shaking hands, hugging or from toilet seats. It can also not be transmitted by tears, sweat, saliva and spitting, urine or faeces (poo).

It is absolutely safe to share objects someone with HIV has touched or used to eat or drink from, and there is no risk of transmission from swimming pools, showers, hot tubs or towels.

Sharing a razor presents a small theoretical risk of transmitting HIV, but sharing razors is never advisable due to the possibility of transmitting bacterial and viral infections including hepatitis B or hepatitis C.

5. 'People with HIV can't have children'

You can have children if you are living with HIV if you are on effective treatment and have an undetectable viral load – the risk of HIV being passed on to the baby is just 0.1%.

Thanks to antenatal screening, treatment to block transmission and caesarean (c-section) delivery, only 0.3% of people with HIV (including people with a higher viral load) passed on HIV to their babies.

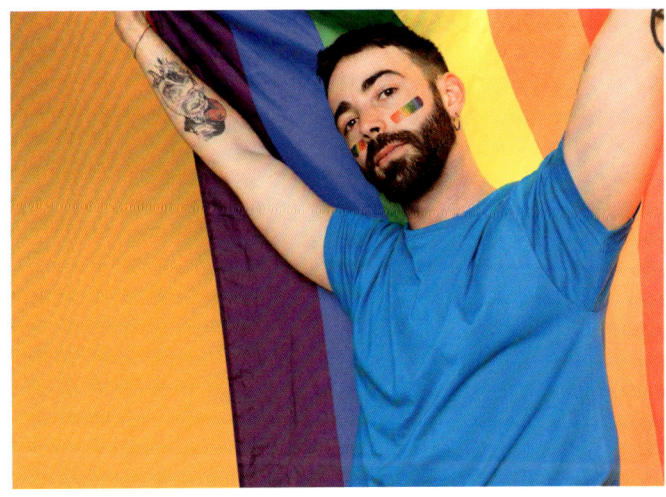

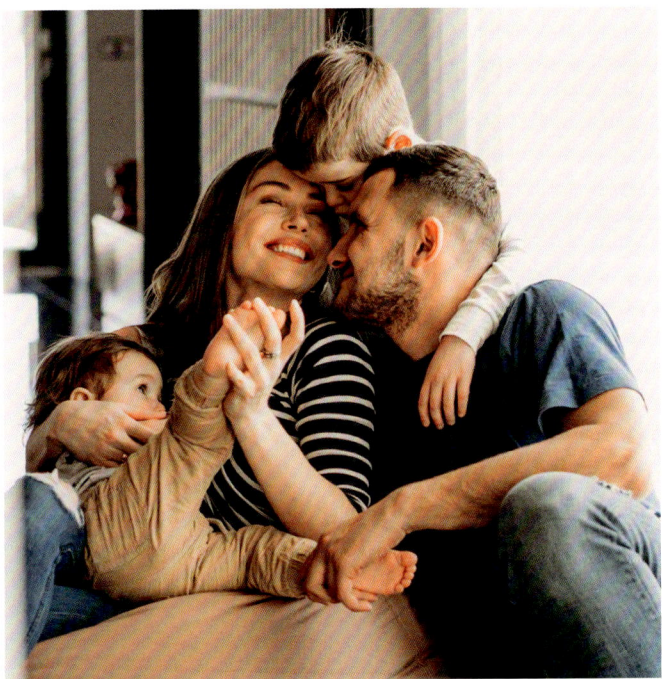

6. 'HIV only affects gay men'

HIV can, and does, affect anyone of any age, sexuality, ethnicity or gender. In the UK, around half of people living with HIV are gay and bi men and the other half are straight people.

Since the start of the epidemic in the 1980s, gay and bisexual men and other men who have sex with men have been the group at highest risk of HIV in the UK. But anyone can be at risk of HIV if they do not protect themselves.

In 2022, the UK Health Security Agency (UKHSA) announced that the number of new HIV diagnoses among heterosexuals is higher than for gay and bisexual men.

Gay and bisexual men are still more impacted by HIV relative to population size, but targeted interventions for this group have led to one of the big success stories of the epidemic.

Late diagnosis of HIV (when someone has been living with HIV unawares for a while) remains high, particularly in those who are of Black African ethnicity, older people, women, and heterosexual men.

7. 'Condoms are the only way to prevent HIV'

Condoms are an effective way to prevent HIV transmission but there's also a pill you can take to protect against HIV.

PrEP (pre-exposure prophylaxis) is a HIV prevention pill taken by HIV-negative people before and after sex that reduces the risk of getting HIV. Taking PrEP before being exposed to HIV means there's enough drug inside you to block HIV if it gets into your body.

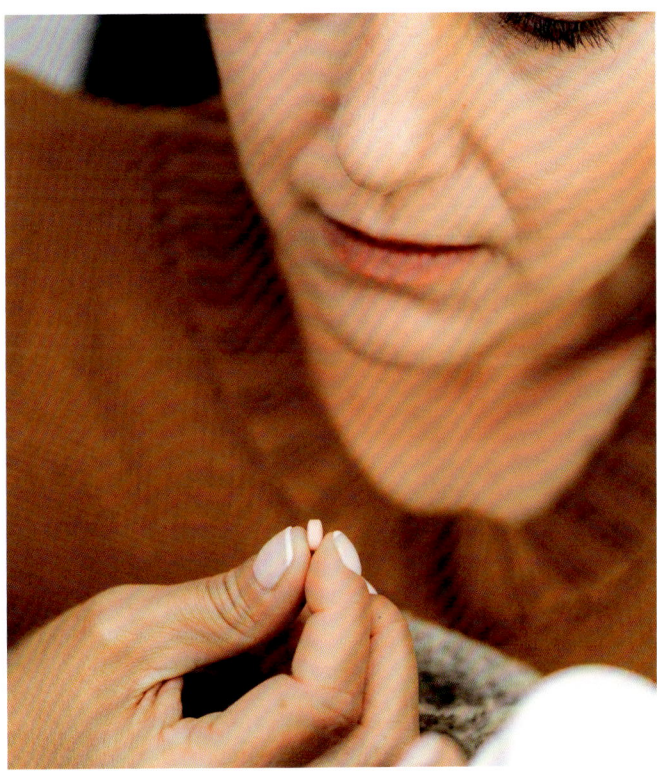

PrEP is available on the NHS.

PrEP is highly effective at preventing HIV. Condoms can help protect you from other STIs or an unplanned pregnancy.

24 October 2023

The above information is reprinted with kind permission from the Terrence Higgins Trust.

© 2024 Terrence Higgins Trust

www.tht.org.uk

An HPV factsheet – everything you need to know

HPV is the most common STI in the world, affecting 80% of the population. Here, Dr Deborah Lee, from Dr Fox Online Pharmacy, addresses the most common issues about the condition.

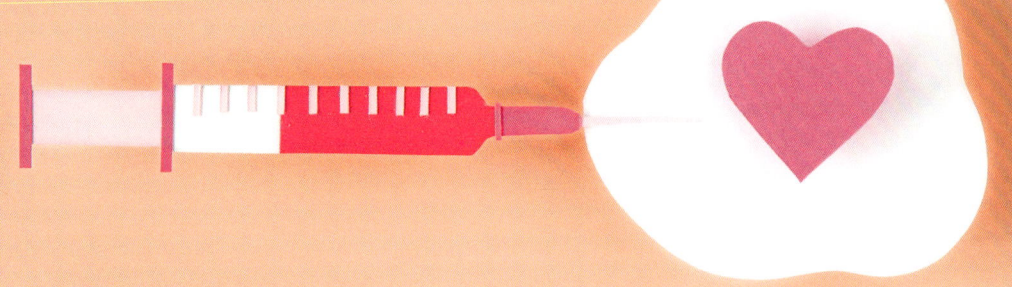

Discussing HPV with a patient in the sexual health clinic is one of the hardest conversations to have. At least with chlamydia, a patient may know how they got the infection, they can be given a successful antibiotic treatment, and afterwards, a test can be taken to show the infection has cleared.

With HPV – the reverse is true. The patient is often mystified as to where it came from, worried their partner has been unfaithful, full of anxiety about living with the infection in the future and being unable to have a test to show whether it is still present or has disappeared.

HPV affects 80% of the population

It's important to try and normalise the situation – they have joined the ranks of the 80% of the population who have it. There's every chance it will disappear by itself within two years. They must not feel ashamed or beat themselves up over it. If there is obvious distress the patient may need a referral for psychosexual counselling.

What is HPV?

HPV stands for human papillomavirus. HPV is the most common STI in the world. By the time we reach the age of 50, 80% of us have encountered the HPV virus, which is shed from the skin and from mucosal surfaces such as the mouth, the vagina, the urethra (the tube that runs down the centre of the penis), and the anal canal.

HPV is a DNA virus. It enters the body through tiny breaches in the skin and reproduces in the basal layers of the epithelium (skin). The virus is clever and often avoids immunological detection by the host, meaning it can persist for long periods, often months or years, and can be difficult to treat. This means the virus has become dormant, and it can stay in this state for 10–20 years, only to reactivate in later life.

HPV statistics

3.2% of women are believed to have high-risk HPV in their cervix in the UK, at any one time.

Estimates suggest 8 in 10 people will be infected with HPV at some stage in their lifetime. But the vast majority will be completely unaware.

What are the types of HPV?

According to the National Library of Medicine, there are over 200 different subtypes of HPV.

- HPV 1, 2, 4, 27 and 57 – cause warts on the skin and the soles of the feet (verrucas). These are a nuisance but do not have malignant potential.
- HPV 6 and 11 – low-risk oncogenic (cancer-causing) subtypes that most often cause anogenital warts.
- HPV 16 and 18 – the most common, high-risk oncogenic subtypes which cause cancerous or precancerous changes on the cervix (the neck of the womb), male and female anogenital regions, and the pharynx (mouth).

Most subtypes of HPV are asymptomatic

It's extremely common for HPV to be present but for the person to be totally unaware of it, and have no symptoms or signs. At present, there are no agreed tests for HPV – apart from in research studies. People only know if they are HPV positive if they develop visible genital warts or have HPV detected with a cervical smear (see below).

HPV and its natural progression

Nine out of 10 cases of HPV disappear by themselves eventually – usually after 12 months or so. The body mounts an antibody response which destroys the virus. But some people, for reasons that are unclear, can have persistent infection with high-risk HPV and hence remain at increased risk of cancer at the affected site – oropharynx (the mouth and throat), vulva, vaginal, penis, or anus.

What is the HPV vaccine?

Three HPV vaccines have been developed which are collectively effective against nine different HPV subtypes.

Three HPV vaccines:

- Gardasil (2006) – protective against HPV 6 and 11, and HPV 16 and 18.
- Cervarix (2007) – protective against HPV 16 and 18.
- Gardasil-9 (2014) – protective against HPV 6, 11, 16, 18, 31, 33, 45, 53 and 58.

Since 2012, Gardasil has been used to immunise school children between the ages of 12 and 13 (year 8). This is because girls and boys need to be vaccinated before they become sexually active.

What do we know about the safety of HPV vaccines?

The HPV vaccines are safe, with very few contraindications.

HPV vaccination is currently not recommended for women during pregnancy, although if a vaccine has been given inadvertently, current data does not show it causes harm to mother or baby. The vaccine can be given during breastfeeding. The most common side effects are redness and pain at the injection site, or headache, although most report no side effects at all.

The schedule for having the HPV vaccine involves having two injections, a first one and a second one, 6 to 24 months later. However, in June 2022, the vaccination used was switched over to Gardasil-9. Anyone up to age 25 is eligible to have Gardasil-9 free on the NHS. Up to age 45, the HPV vaccine can be purchased and administered privately.

How does the HIV vaccine work?

The HPV vaccine used proteins which act as virus-like particles (VLPs). These trick the body into thinking it has been in contact with the HPV virus, and hence antibodies are produced. In the future, if the HPV virus does enter the body, the immune system remembers it has seen this before and quickly produces antibodies which destroy the virus before it can become established.

What is the vaccine efficacy

The HPV vaccine is highly effective at preventing cervical cancer. HPV is believed to cause 99% of cases of cervical cancer. The HPV vaccination programme started in 2008. Over the following 11 years, rates of cervical cancer in those in their early 20s, who were given the vaccine aged 12 or 13, dropped by 90%. Estimates suggest that during this time the HPV vaccine prevented 450 cases of cervical cancer, and 17,200 cases of precancerous changes on the cervix.

Other studies have shown that the HPV vaccination is effective in preventing HPV infection, genital warts and high-grade precancerous changes in the cervix.

Even though the vaccine is highly effective, women should still have regular cervical smears. The currently available vaccines do not protects against all HPV subtypes.

Understanding HPV transmission

HPV is transmitted by skin-to-skin contact or via skin-to-mucosal surfaces. This means it is spread by touching, and petting, and does not necessarily require sexual intercourse.

It is spread by all types of sexual activity/genital-to-genital contact – peno-vaginal, peno-oral and peno-anal sex. It is not spread in blood or semen. But it can be transmitted for example, on fingers, the outside of a condom, gloves, sex toys, and tubes of lubricant.

It is not spread in blood or semen.

HPV can live under the fingernails, meaning it's possible to infect yourself!

This has been demonstrated in those who have never had sex and in children.

HPV is very infectious. Most people are unaware they are HPV positive. Hence it is most often passed on completely inadvertently. 70% of sexual partners of anyone who has an HPV infection are likely to become infected.

Babies can become infected after passage through an infected birth canal. This can cause polyps on their vocal cords – juvenile papillomatosis.

It is so common to be HPV-positive that we need to regard it as a normal part of life. It's important to try not to be ashamed if you find you are HPV positive or develop warts. 80% of those aged 50 have been exposed to the HPV virus at some stage in their lives.

The best way to protect yourself from HPV is to have an HPV vaccination.

How can a woman in a long-term relationship get HPV?

Being married or in a long-term relationship does not prevent a woman from being infected with HPV. Many women erroneously think they cannot be at risk of HPV – but this is not the case. HPV is so common – every woman has to consider herself at risk. It also does not mean she or her partner has been unfaithful.

The virus can be present in the body for a long time – even years – before it is detected. The woman may well have been infected before she met her current partner – her husband. She could have even become infected the first time she had sex. The HPV virus can become dormant and rest inside the body for many years, even decades, before it becomes active.

Her husband may have infected her when they met, however long ago that was, but neither of them knew until now.

Sadly, women can get infected when receiving medical care. In one study 17.9% of gynaecological equipment tested positive for HPV, with contamination being nearly three times higher in private clinics than in hospital clinics. Infected sites included sterile gloves and colposcopy equipment.

It's important to be sensitive as she could also have been sexually assaulted in the past or raped.

The woman might work in a healthcare setting and have picked up HPV at work, on her fingers, by touching an infected piece of equipment and inadvertently passed it to the vulva or vagina, perhaps when wiping herself in the toilet.

It's true that either she or her husband could have recently had – or have had – other sexual partners. But this may not be the case at all. If a woman does test positive for HPV, it's important to reassure her that this does not mean her partner has been unfaithful.

What are the symptoms of HPV in women?

Most often, HPV does not cause any symptoms. The majority of women (and men) with HPV are unaware they have it.

However, HPV causes genital warts – which are small bumps, often rough to the touch, which can be darkly pigmented or flesh-coloured, and are found on the genitalia – the vulva, vagina, cervix, penis or anal skin. They may not cause symptoms or are sometimes itchy.

HPV is routinely tested for when a woman has a cervical smear. This may be the only way a woman knows she carries the virus. If this is high-risk HPV, and she has abnormal cells on the smear, she will be referred to the colposcopy clinic, where her cervix can be examined in greater detail and biopsies taken. If she is high-risk HPV positive but has a normal smear, she will simply be asked to have a repeat smear in one year's time.

HPV also causes anogenital malignancies – vulval, vaginal, penile and anal cancers. The precursor to these cancers are precancerous changes in the skin called intraepithelial neoplasia – known respectively as vulval intraepithelial neoplasia (VIN), vaginal intraepithelial neoplasia (VaIN), penile intraepithelial neoplasia (PIN) and anal intraepithelial neoplasia (AIN).

These conditions present as small discoloured, raised or sometimes ulcerated, patches on the anogenital regions, which can be itchy and sometimes bleed. They can be flesh-coloured, red, pink or brown, and the skin is often thickened.

Although HPV is a causative factor, the herpes simplex virus, a weakened immune system, and smoking are also implicated.

When to seek medical help

If a woman notices any usual skin patches or changes in the genital region it's vital to see her GP or go to the Sexual Health Clinic. The diagnosis is made on a biopsy. As with all medical conditions, getting a prompt diagnosis gives the best chance of a good outcome.

HPV testing is not routinely offered on the NHS. This is because the diagnosis can cause anxiety and distress and there is no current way to eradicate it from the body. HPV is tested for when cervical smears are taken. Women are not recommended to get tested for HPV under the age of 25.

Can HPV be cured?

There are no current treatments for HPV. Any lesions it causes, such as genital warts or changes to the cervix are treated, to get rid of the abnormality and help prompt the immune system to produce a better antibody response.

Don't smoke – smoking is a well-recognised risk factor for cervical cancer. Noxious chemicals in cigarette smoke impair the immune response to cervical HPV infection. Giving up smoking can lead to the resolution of abnormal cells on the cervix. Smoking allows the virus to grow and divide more rapidly. If a woman has an abnormal smear, stopping smoking will greatly improve her chances of recovery.

Genital warts are treated with a range of different options including cryotherapy, topical treatment such as podophyllin, or the use of Imiquimod (a cream which stimulates the antibody response). They can be surgically removed using electrocautery or laser.

How often do people infected with HPV develop cancer?

The majority of people infected with HPV will never know they are infected and will never develop cancer.

90% of women with HPV will become clear of the infection within two years of being infected.

In the 10% with ongoing infections, only a small % age will go on to develop abnormal smears.

High-risk HPV is said to cause 3% of cancers in females, and 2% of cancers in males.

Overall, persistent HPV virus infection is thought to be responsible for 5% of cancers.

HPV in men

HPV affects men just as it does women. It causes genital warts on the penis and in the anus and around the anal margins. It can cause PIN and AIN, which can be low-grade or high-grade and can progress to penile or anal cancers.

How long can HPV be dormant?

No-one is quite sure of the answer to this question. HPV infection has a long latent phase which can last 10–20 years before the development of cervical cancer occurs. After this time, if HPV is detected it's hard to say if this is the same infection or a new infection with a different subtype.

Final thoughts on HPV

It's a sobering thought that most of us will become infected with HPV during our lifetime. What we can do is ensure our young people are protected by making sure they are vaccinated before they become sexually active.

Meanwhile, the burden of HPV exists, and we all have to live with it. There should be no shame or stigma attached to a diagnosis of HPV. Even those who have never had sexual intercourse can have HPV. We have to learn to live with HPV, like we have to accept other common infections like Covid-19.

27 February 2023

Design

Design a poster either promoting the HPV vaccine, or to persuade women to have a cervical screening appointment.

The above information is reprinted with kind permission from Open Access Government.
© 2024 Adjacent Digital Politics Ltd

www.openaccessgovernment.org

STIs through the centuries

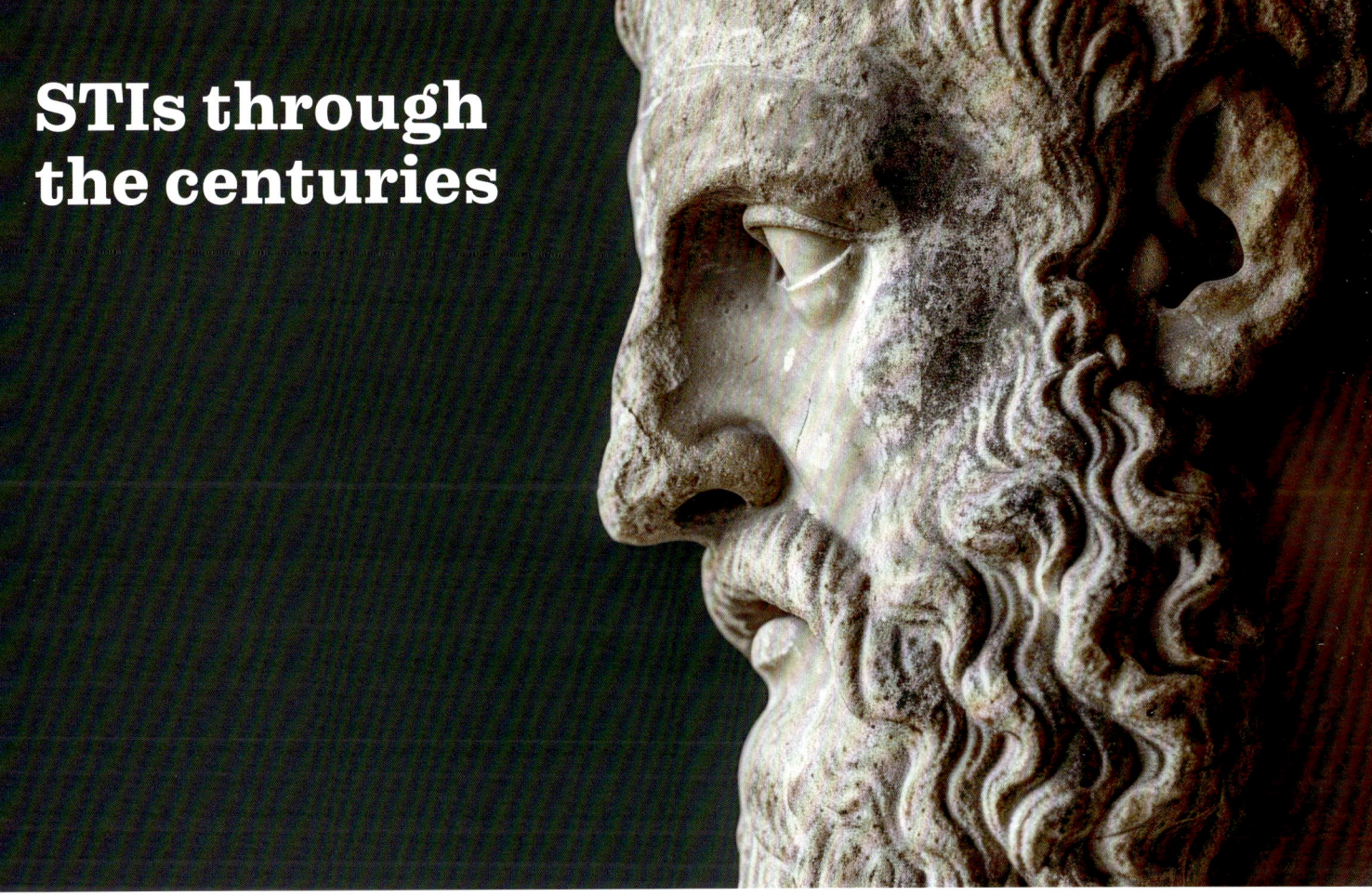

In England, data produced by the UKHSA shows that year after year new diagnoses of sexually transmitted infections (STIs) remain high and, between 2021 and 2022, diagnoses of gonorrhoea and infectious syphilis increased by 50% and 15% respectively.

In this article we will explore the rising tide of STIs across the eons, how ancient Greeks feared the killer 'scorpions and serpents' in semen, and how goat's milk was thought to be a curative for sexual ailments.

The ancient world

The Greek and Roman Period (5th century BCE – 4th century CE)

Over 2,400 years ago the ancient Greeks and Romans were documenting their complex sexual networks and their sexual health.

Love and relationships in the time of The Minotaur and Medusa were not without their dangers. It is recorded that Pasiphae, the wife of King Minos of Crete, used a goat's bladder as a condom as the King's semen was said to contain 'scorpions and serpents' that killed his mistresses.

And thanks to the ancient Greek physician Hippocrates, referred to as the Father of Medicine, we have some insights into the prevalence of diseases resembling STIs through his descriptions of clinical cases.

Writings from the *Hippocratic Corpus* describe what might be acute gonorrhoea as 'strangury', which is thought to be caused by indulgences in the pleasures of Venus.

The name gonorrhoea is as ancient as its descriptions, being coined by another Greek doctor before 200 CE, Galen refers to gonorrhoea as 'an unwanted discharge of semen'.

Medieval era

The Islamic Golden Age (8th – 14th centuries)

The Persian Rhazes (865-925 CE), a doctor and director of hospitals of what would become Baghdad, describes genital ulcers and what is thought to be gonorrhoea in his text *Continens* with the treatment at the time being the slow introduction of goat's or breast milk to the infection.

These early writings included the transmission of diseases through sexual contact, laying the foundation for future understanding from other Persian doctors such as Aly Abbas who would diagnose and record infections from urethral discharge, burning sensations while urinating and thick discoloured discharge.

European Middle Ages (4th – 14th centuries)

STIs in the Middle Ages were often linked to moral judgements. The term 'venereal diseases' emerged in the Middle English period between 1150 and 1500, named after Venus, the goddess of love, the term venereal disease nods back to Hippocrates and, while misogynistic in origin, emphasises the connection of infections to sexual activity.

Renaissance and Early Modern period

The Renaissance (14th – 17th centuries)

The Renaissance promoted the rediscovery of classical philosophy, literature and art but is also believed to have coincided with either the introduction or discovery of syphilis in Europe.

The origin of syphilis in Europe is highly debated by academics. Some argue that evidence from combined paleopathology and molecular analyses suggests the increased movement of people across the continent, and between this and other continents encouraged the spread.

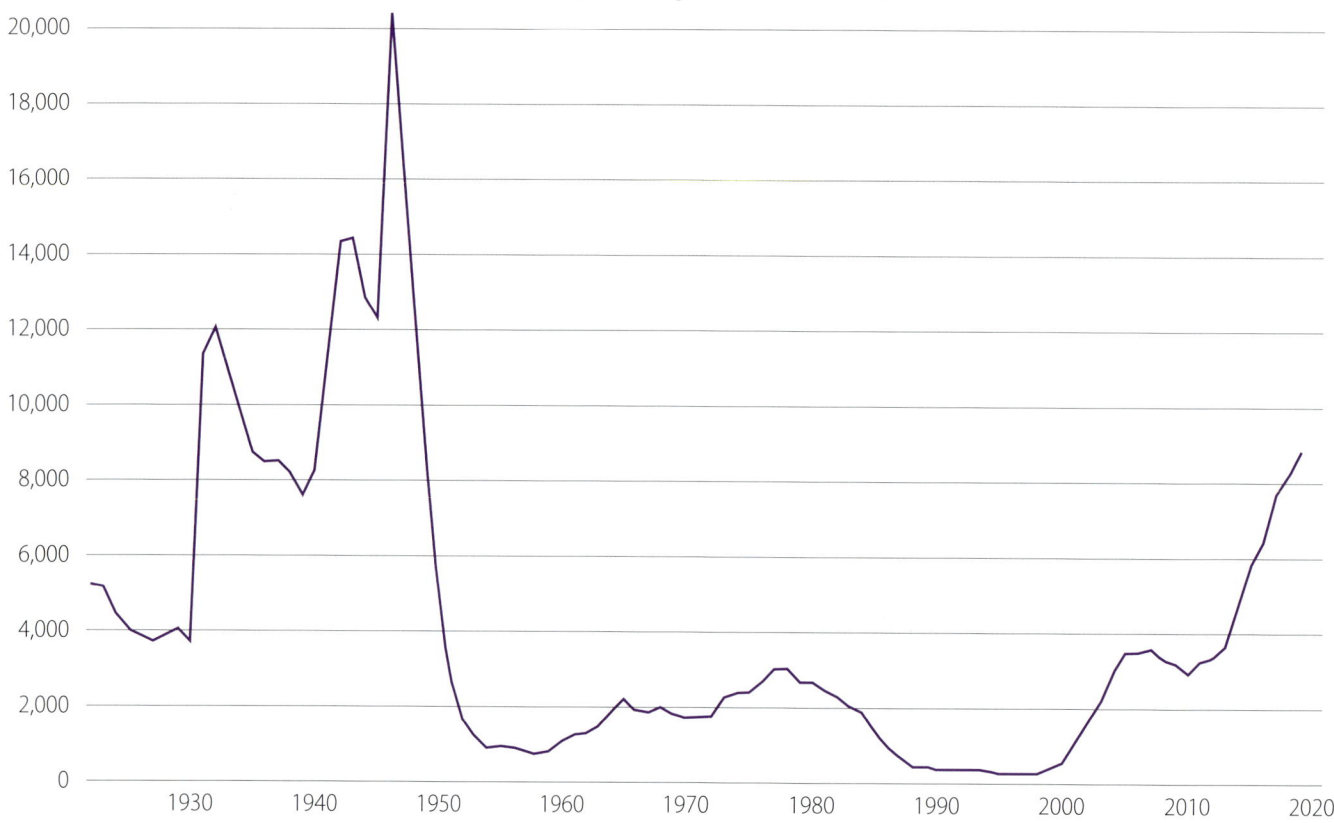

*UK data may not always include data from England, Wales, Scotland and Northern Ireland due to availability of surveillance data. Data includes diagnoses of primary, secondary and early latent syphilis. UK data for 2020 to 2024 are not currently available.
Source: UKHSA

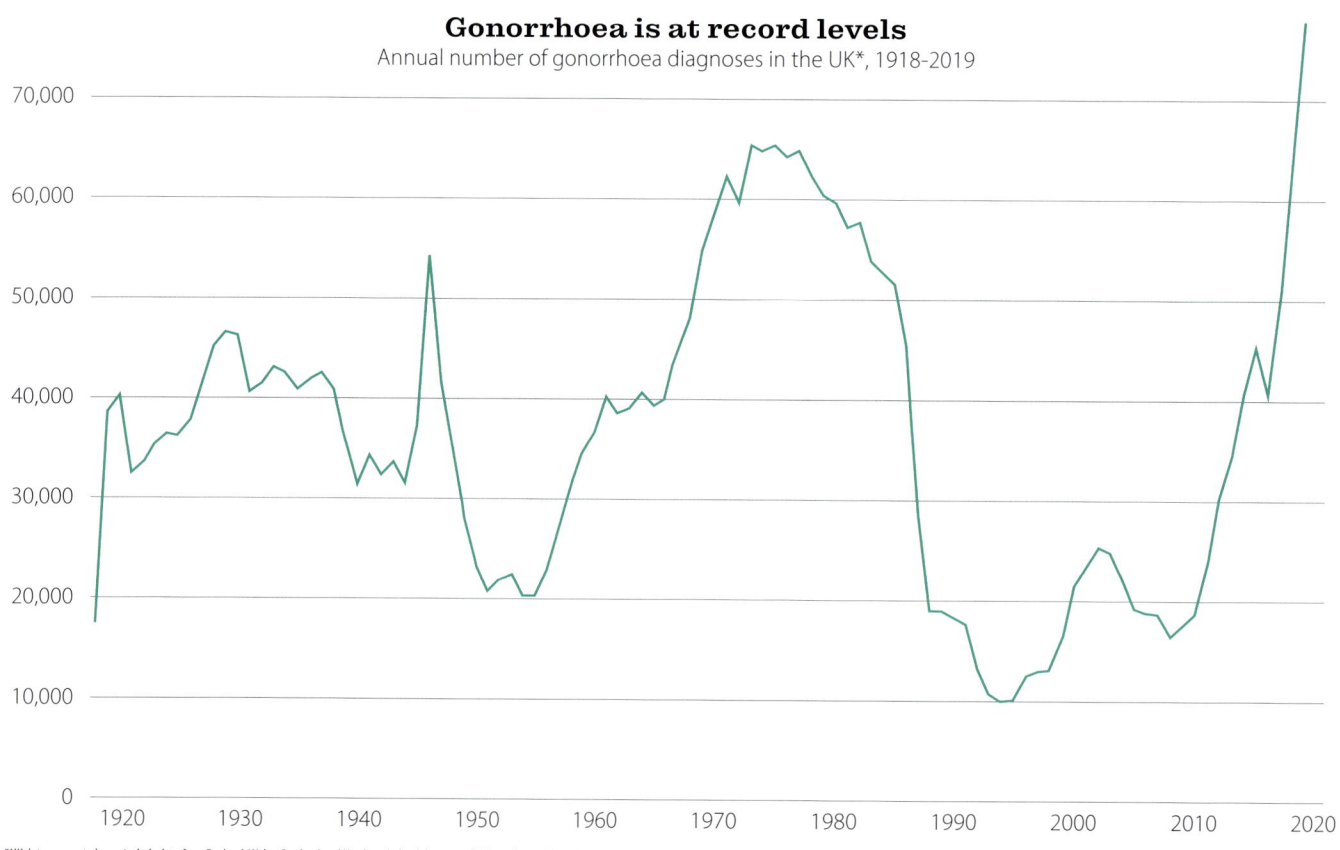

*UK data may not always include data from England, Wales, Scotland and Northern Ireland due to availability of surveillance data. UK data for 2020 to 2024 are not currently available.
Source: UKHSA

issues: Sexual Health & STIs — Chapter 3: STIs

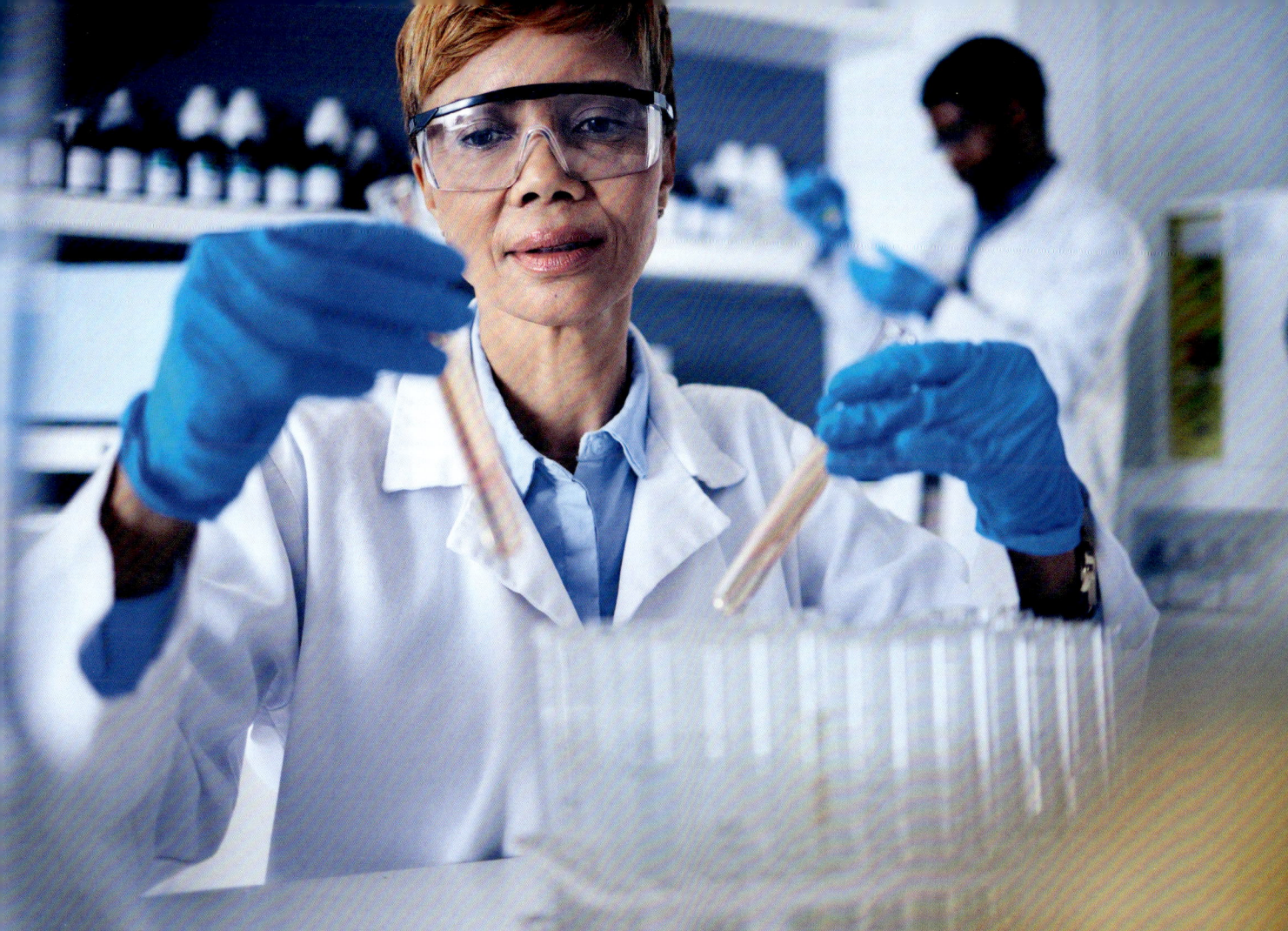

19th century

The Germ Theory

Advances in microscopy allowed for the identification of specific pathogens and in the 19th century was a turning point in which microorganisms such as bacteria, viruses, fungi and parasites were accepted as the cause of disease, illness and infection.

Germ theory saw the beginning of an era with a more scientific approach to understanding and treating infections, including STIs.

Germ theory allowed for a better understanding of transmission routes from person to person and the development of treatments and the discovery of antibiotics, such as penicillin in the mid-20th century, revolutionised the treatment of STIs, including syphilis and gonorrhoea.

Resurgence

In 2022, gonorrhoea diagnoses were the highest they have been since records began in 1918, and syphilis diagnoses were the highest they have been since 1948.

The increase in diagnoses will in part be due to the success of an increase in testing and detection of more infections, but the scale of the increase in diagnoses in recent years strongly suggests that there is more transmission of STIs within the population driven by various factors such as decreasing condom use.

UKHSA, and other public health bodies charged with monitoring and charting rises and falls in STIs have been doing so in the UK since 1918.

The future of sexual health

Sexually transmitted infections have been around for aeons, but that doesn't mean they're here to stay. Discoveries and innovations such as Pre-Exposure Prophylaxis (PrEP) have been used to dramatically reduce the risk of getting HIV (human immunodeficiency virus), and effective HIV treatment now means that those who adhere to their medication cannot pass on the virus, known as undetectable = untransmittible (U=U).

In the UK, the British Association for Sexual Health and HIV is working with UKHSA on new guidance to inform the prescribing of doxycycline post exposure prophylaxis (Doxy-PEP) for the prevention of bacterial STIs such as syphilis.

And in the UK, the Joint Committee on Vaccination and Immunisation have recently advised the Government on the targeted use of the 4CMenB vaccine for the prevention of gonorrhoea.

13 March 2024

The above information is reprinted with kind permission from DEPARTMENT.

© Crown Copyright 2024

This information is licensed under the Open Government Licence v3.0

To view this licence, visit http://www.nationalarchives.gov.uk/doc/open-government-licence/

www.gov.uk

Useful Websites

Useful websites

www.adph.org.uk

www.brook.org.uk

www.devonsexualhealth.nhs.uk

www.gov.uk

www.healthforteens.co.uk

www.hiddenstrength.com

www.independent.co.uk

www.nhs.uk

www.openaccessgovernment.org

www.psychologytoday.com

www.sh24.org.uk

www.tht.org.uk

www.topdoctors.co.uk

www.ukhsa.blog.gov.uk

www.young.scot

www.yourgenome.org

Where can I find help?

Below are some telephone numbers, email addresses, and websites of agencies or charities that can offer support or advice if you, or someone you know, needs it.

NHS
NHS 111 by dialling 111 (England and Wales, all-age)
NHS 24 call 08454 242424 (Scotland, all-age)

NHS Health for Teens
www.healthforteens.co.uk

Brook
www.brook.org.uk

National Sexual Health Helpline
Helpline: 0300 123 7123

ChildLine
Helpline: 0800 11 11
www.childline.org.uk

Family Planning Association
Helpline: 0300 123 7123 (Mon-Fri, 9am-8pm; Saturday and Sunday, 11am-4pm)
www.fpa.org.uk

Terrence Higgins Trust
Helpline: 0808 802 1221
www.tht.org.uk

Sexwise
www.sexwise.org.uk

MSI Reproduction
www.msichoices.org.uk

Glossary

AIDS
Acquired immune deficiency syndrome. AIDS is a potentially fatal illness. It develops at the most advanced stage of HIV.

Cervical cancer
Cancer that develops in a woman's cervix (the entrance to the womb from the vagina). In its early stages it often has no symptoms. Symptoms can include unusual vaginal bleeding which can occur after sex, in between periods or after menopause. The NHS offers a national screening programme; a 'smear test' for all women over 24 years old.

Condoms
A thin rubber (latex) sleeve worn on the penis. When used correctly, condoms are the only form of contraception that protect against pregnancy and STIs. They are 98% effective – this means that two out of 100 women using male condoms as contraception will become pregnant in one year. You can get free condoms from sexual health clinics and some GP surgeries.

Contraception
Anything which prevents conception, or pregnancy, from taking place. 'Barrier methods', such as condoms, work by stopping sperm from reaching an egg during intercourse and are also effective in preventing sexually transmitted infections (STIs). Hormonal methods such as the contraceptive pill change the way a woman's body works to prevent an egg from being fertilised. Emergency contraception, commonly known as the 'morning-after pill', is used after unprotected sex to prevent a fertilised egg from becoming implanted in the womb.

Contraceptive implant
A small flexible tube about the size of a matchstick inserted by a doctor under the skin of a female's upper arm. The device releases hormones to prevent the ovaries from releasing eggs. Lasts for three years, but can be removed before then if the woman decided she wants to get pregnant.

Contraceptive injections
An injection offers eight to 12 weeks protection against pregnancy, but not from sexually transmitted diseases (approx. 99% effective). It works by thickening the mucus in the cervix, which stops sperm reaching the egg, and it also thins the lining of the womb so that an egg can't implant itself there.

Diaphragms
A rubber dome-shaped device worn inside the vagina which creates a seal against the walls of the vagina. It must be inserted before sexual intercourse and must remain in places for up to six to eight hours afterwards. The diaphragm does not provide protection from sexually transmitted diseases.

Emergency contraception
Sometimes referred to as the 'morning-after pill', this is a form of emergency contraception which can be taken by girls within 72 hours after unprotected sex (although preferably within the first 24 hours). It should not be used as a regular method of contraceptive. It is available across the counter at chemists or from your local GP, family planning clinic or sexual health clinic.

Female condom
Sometimes known as a femidom, a female condom is worn inside the vagina during sex to prevent pregnancy. They're a barrier method of contraception, protecting against pregnancy as well as STIs. If used correctly they are 95% effective.

HIV
Human Immunodeficiency. A virus passed-on through certain bodily fluids such as infected blood, genital fluids, breast milk and semen. It cannot be passed through kissing or touching. HIV attacks the cells of the immune system, making it hard for the body to fight infections. Immediately after contracting HIV, a person may experience flu-like symptoms which will then disappear. At later stages of infection, symptoms include fatigue, weight loss, sores in the mouth and pneumonia. HIV can, eventually, progress to AIDS.

HPV vaccination
The vaccine is effective at stopping people getting the high-risk types of HPV that cause cancer, including most cervical cancers and some anal, genital, mouth and throat (head and neck) cancers. In England, all boys and girls aged 12 to 13 years are routinely offered the first HPV vaccination when they're in Year 8 at school. The second dose is offered 6 to 24 months after the first dose.

Safe sex
Being safe with sex means caring for both your own health, and the health of your partner. Being safe protects you from getting or passing on STIs and from unplanned pregnancy.

Sexual health
Taking care of your sexual health means more than being free from sexually transmissible infections (STIs) or not having to face an unplanned pregnancy. It also means taking responsibility for your body, your health, your partner's health and your decisions about sex.

Sexually transmitted infections (STIs)
A sexually transmitted infection (STIs), also referred to as sexually transferred diseases (STDs), is a bacterial or viral infection that is spread through sexual contact. This doesn't just mean vaginal/anal sexual intercourse, but also oral sex (licking/sucking on someone's genitals) and sexual touching (skin-to-skin contact). Using condoms are the best way of avoiding STIs. Although STIs are treatable, if left unchecked and untreated they may cause serious damage to long-term health, such as infertility. The most common STI in the UK is chlamydia.

The pill
A tablet taken each day, at the same time, by girls to prevent pregnancy. The pill contains hormones that prevent the ovaries from releasing an egg. It only protects against pregnancy and not STIs.

Index

A
age of consent 11, 13
AIDS and HIV 3, 20, 25, 28, 31–35
alcohol 11, 14
assault, sexual 5

B
birth control *see* contraception

C
chlamydia 5, 23, 26–27, 28
communication, good 10, 12, 13
condoms 14, 16, 20, 30
confidentiality 5
consent 10–11, 13
contraception 15–22 *see also* condoms
    emergency 4, 5, 14, 18, 21
    history of 2
    types 16–18
    where to get 19, 22

D
drugs 11, 14

E
emergency help 4–5, 18, 20, 21

F
funding for sexual health 27

G
genital hygiene 8–9
genital warts 28, 29, 38
gonorrhoea 23, 25, 26–27, 28, 39–41

H
HIV/AIDS 3, 20, 25, 28, 31–35
HPV (human papillomavirus) 7, 28–29, 36–38

L
learning disabilities 11

M
morning-after pill 14, 19, 21
mycoplasma genitalium 29
myths 14, 30, 34–35

P
pharmacies 21, 22
pill, birth control 5, 14, 16–17, 19, 21, 22
pornography 14
pregnancy, unplanned 4, 14, 21
pressure to have sex 5, 10–11
pubic lice 29
'pull out' method 14, 30

R
rates of STIs 25, 26–27
readiness for sex 12, 13
responsibility and safety 12, 13

S
scabies 29
sexual health check-ups 6
sexual health services (SHS) 2–3
smear tests 7, 38
STIs (sexually transmitted infections)
    contraception and 15
    emergency help 4–5
    getting tested 6, 20, 23, 25
    history of 3, 39–41
    people at risk 14, 25
    preventing 28–29, 30, 31
    symptoms and treatment 23, 24, 25
    types 28–29
symptoms
    HIV/AIDS 32–33
    HPV (human papillomavirus) 36, 38
    STIs 23, 24
syphilis 25, 26, 29, 39–41

T
teenage pregnancy 2–3
testing
    HIV/AIDS 31
    STIs 4, 20, 23, 25
transmission
    HIV/AIDS 32, 34–35
    HPV (human papillomavirus) 37–38
treatment
    HIV/AIDS 31, 33, 34
    HPV (human papillomavirus) 38
    STIs 23, 25
trichomonas 29

U
unprotected sex 4–5, 14, 21

V
vaccines, HPV 36–37

Y
yeast infection 29